Inflammation and Angiogenesis

Domenico Ribatti

Inflammation and Angiogenesis

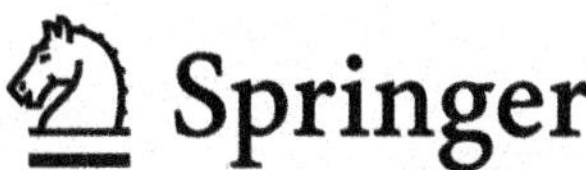 Springer

Domenico Ribatti
Department of Biomedical Sciences
Neurosciences and Sensory Organs
University of Bari Medical School
Bari, Italy

ISBN 978-3-319-88604-6   ISBN 978-3-319-68448-2   (eBook)
https://doi.org/10.1007/978-3-319-68448-2

This Springer imprint is published by Springer Nature
The registered company is Springer International Publishing AG
The registered company address is: Gewerbestrasse 11, 6330 Cham, Switzerland

Abstract

Both innate and adaptive immune cells are involved in the mechanisms of endothelial cell proliferation, migration, and activation, through the production and release of a large spectrum of proangiogenic mediators. These may create the specific microenvironment that favors an increased rate of tissue vascularization. In this book, I will focus on the immune cell component of the angiogenic process in inflammation and tumor growth. The link between chronic inflammation and tumorigenesis was first proposed by Rudolf Virchow in 1863 after the observation that infiltrating leukocytes are a hallmark of tumors and first established a causative connection between the lymphoreticular infiltrate at sites of chronic inflammation and the development of cancer. Surgeons have long described the tendency of tumors to recur in healing resection margin, and it has been reported that wound healing environment provides an opportunistic matrix for tumor growth. Tumors were described by Harold Dvorak as wounds that never heal.

As angiogenesis is the result of a net balance between the activities exerted by positive and negative regulators, I will also provide information on some antiangiogenic properties of immune cells that may be utilized for a potential pharmacological use as antiangiogenic agents in inflammation as well as in cancer.

Contents

Chapter 1
Introduction

Angiogenesis (new vessel formation) occurs during embryo development and in postnatal life, cyclically in the female genital system and in wound repair. In these situations, it is limited in time and the result of an equilibrium between the activator and the inhibitor systems that together keep the microcirculation in a quiescent state, with very low proliferation and turnover of the endothelial cells (Fig. 1.1).

Tumor angiogenesis is uncontrolled and unlimited in time, and characterized by a 30/40-fold proliferative activity of endothelial cells (Ribatti and Vacca 2008) It is essential for tumor progression in the form of growth, invasion and metastasis because these develop through the transition from the avascular to the vascular phase. The avascular phase appears to correspond to the histopathological picture presented by a small colony of neoplastic cells that reaches a steady state before it proliferates and becomes rapidly invasive. In this scenario, metabolites and catabolites are transferred by simple diffusion through the surrounding tissue, and the cells at the periphery of the tumor continue to reproduce, whereas those in the deeper portion die away. If the vascular phase is dependent on angiogenesis and release of angiogenic factors, acquisition of angiogenic capability through the so called "angiogenic switch" (Fig. 1.2) (Hanahan and Folkman 1996; Ribatti et al. 2007) can be seen as an expression of the progression from neoplastic transformation to tumor growth and metastasis (Ribatti et al. 2006a). Practically all solid tumors, including those of the colon, lung, breast, cervix, bladder, prostate and pancreas, progress through these two phases. The role of angiogenesis in the growth and survival of leukemias and other hematological malignancies has only become evident since 1994 thanks to a series of studies demonstrating that progression in several forms is clearly related to their degree of angiogenesis (Vacca and Ribatti 2006).

The tumor microenvironment is characterized by adverse pathophysiological conditions, especially hypoxia. Hypoxia regulates the expression of many genes under the transcriptional control of hypoxia inducible factors 1α and 2α (HIF1α and HIF2α), which heterodimerize with HIF1β and bind to the hypoxia response element (HRE) (Kaluz et al. 2008). Hypoxia drives pro-inflammatory signaling mediated by HIF and NFkB. The resultant inflammation increases the mass and the

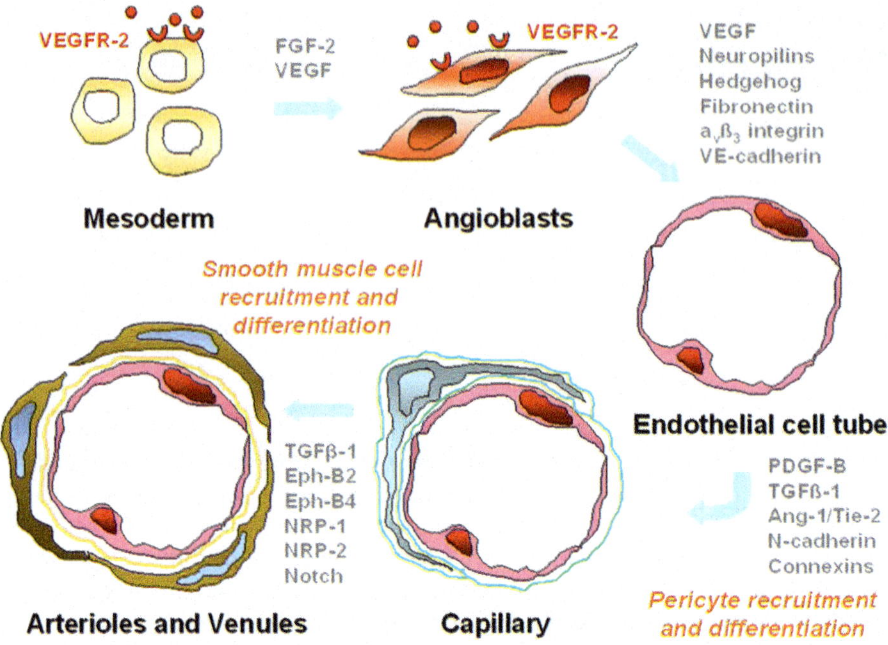

Fig. 1.1 The earliest blood vessels in the embryo originate from mesodermal cells that are specified into angioblasts most likely in response to fibroblast growth factor-2 (FGF-2) and vascular endothelial growth factor (VEGF) signals. Angioblasts begin to differentiate into endothelial cells and assemble into tubes, as the result of VEGF signals from surrounding tissues and the expression of intercellular and cell-matrix adhesion molecules. Endothelial cell tubes are soon stabilized by pericytes recruited from the surrounding mesenchyme to form early capillaries. In microvessels, platelet derived growth factor (PDGF) and transforming growth factor beta 1 (TGFß1) signals are involved in the recruitment of pericytes. In larger vessels, arterioles and venules, the vascular wall is made up of endothelial cells and smooth muscle cells, which are recruited mainly through the Tie-2 and Angiopoietin-1 (Ang-1) receptor-ligand pair, although Neuropilins and Notch pathway are also involved in mural cell formation. Ephrin-B2 and Ephrin-B4 are implicated in arterial and venous endothelial cell specialization, respectively (Reproduced from Ribatti et al. 2009)

metabolic demand of the tissue and triggers the release of pro-angiogenic signals from leukocytes, endothelial cells, and from the extracellular matrix, and remodels the extracellular matrix to facilitate vessel growth (Fig. 1.3). Moreover, hypoxia plays a significant role in determining the tumor response to therapy and influencing the metastatic potential of tumors. Finally, hypoxia may affect cancer stem cells (CSCs) generation and maintenance through the upregulation of HIFs (Baumann et al. 2008; Hill et al. 2009).

The stroma plays a major role in revering differentiated cells towards a dedifferentiated phenotype. This is one of the mechanisms generating CSCs (Hanahan and Weinberg 2011). CSCs amount to around 1–25% of the total viable tumor cell population (Hill et al. 2009), but they are believed to be the cells that must be completely eliminated to obtain tumor control (Baumann et al. 2008). CSCs are often

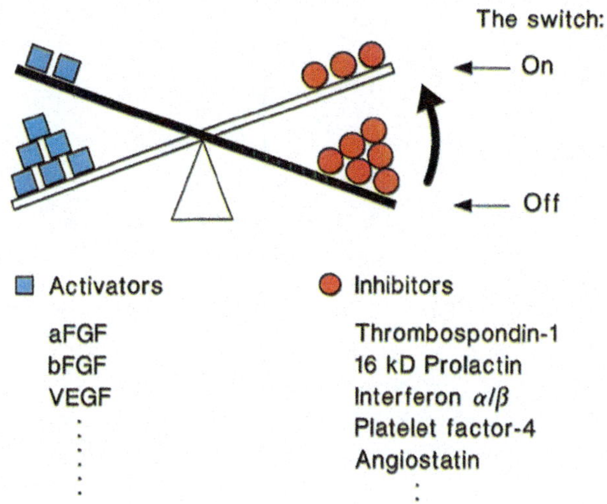

Fig. 1.2 The balance hypothesis of the angiogenic switch. The normally quiescent vasculature can be activated to angiogenesis, a morphogenic process controlled by an angiogenic switch mechanism. Changes in the relative balance of inducers and inhibitors of angiogenesis can activate the switch. In some tissues, the absence of angiogenesis inducers may keep the switch off, while in others the angiogenesis inducers are present but held in check by higher levels of angiogenesis inhibitors. Thus, either reducing the inhibitor concentration, e.g., for thrombospondin-1 (TSP-1), by loss of a tumor suppressor gene; or increasing the activator levels, e.g., for induction of vascular endothelial growth factor (VEGF), by hypoxia, can each change the balance and activate the switch, leading to the growth of new blood vessels (Reproduced from Hanahan and Folkman 1996)

responsible for resistance to anti-angiogenic therapy, as occurs in breast cancer in which the administration of sunitinib and bevacizumab induces tumor hypoxia, increasing the CSC population (Conley et al. 2012).

The tumor microenvironment is a complex system of many cell types, including endothelial cells and their precursors, pericytes, smooth-muscle cells, fibroblasts, neutrophils, eosinophils, basophils, mast cells, T, B and natural killer lymphocytes, and antigen-presenting cells, such as macrophages and dendritic cells, which communicate through a complex network of intercellular signaling pathways that are mediated by surface adhesion molecules, cytokines and their receptors (Fig. 1.4) (Ribatti et al. 2006b). Tumor angiogenesis result not only from the interaction of cancer cells with endothelial cells, but surrounding inflammatory cells have also a crucial role in directiong the neoformation of blood vessels.

A peculiar type of microenevironment is the bone marrow, considered a source of endothelial precursor cells able that participate in the growth of blood vessels during postnatal vasculogenesis as well as in the angiogenic process. Vasculogenesis, originally described as embryonic blood vessel formation from the endothelial precursor cells (EPCs), is also referred to as the formation of new vessels from EPCs in postnatal life (Fig. 1.5). Vasculogenesis leads to the formation of the first major intra-embryonic blood vessels, such as the dorsal aorta and the cardinal veins, and to the formation of the primary vascular plexus in the yolk sac.

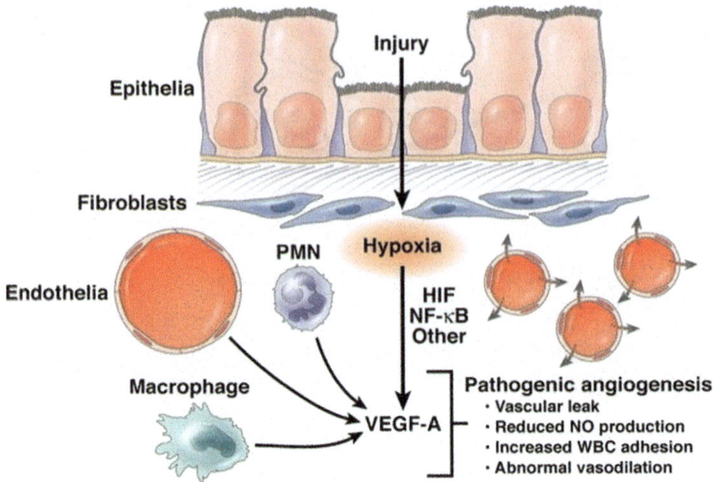

Fig. 1.3 Contributions of inflammation and hypoxia to angiogenesis. Inflammation and hypoxia each contribute to angiogenesis during pathogenesis of inflammatory bowel disease (IBD), partly by induction of vascular endothelial growth factor-A (VEGF-A) expression in multiple cell types that include submucosal fibroblasts, macrophages, neutrophils (PMNs), and endothelial cells. VEGF-A-induced angiogenesis is likely to be pathogenic and result in abnormal vessel formation and poorly functioning vasculature (Reproduced from Glover and Colgan 2011)

With the onset of embryonic circulation, these primary vessels have to be remodeled into arteries and veins in order to develop a functional vascular loop. Remodeling of the primary vascular plexus into a more mature vascular system is thought to occur by a process termed angiogenesis (Fig. 1.5). The term angiogenesis, applied to the formation of capillaries from pre-existing vessels, i.e., capillaries and post-capillary venules, is based on endothelial sprouting microvascular growth.

Bone marrow derived endothelial cells (BMDECs) are involved in promoting indirectly the vascular growth through the expression of angiogenic factors in the site where the neovascularization occurs (Ziegelhoeffer 2004) CXCR4 is highly expressed by BMDECs and is involved in their mobilization and homing. CXCL12 expression is also regulated by VEGF directly. VEGF stimulate the expression of CXCL12 in perivascular cells and the latter attracts CXCR4-positive circulating cells. Blocking VEGF receptor-1 (VEGFR-1) reduces the number of recruited perivascular cells in tumors, suggesting that the effect of VEGF could involve VEGFR-1 (Hattori et al. 2001).

Multiple myeloma is an example of a tumor in which signals from this microenvironment play a critical role in maintaining plasma cell growth, migration and survival (Ribatti et al. 2006b). Reciprocal positive and negative interactions between plasma cells and bone marrow stromal cells (BMSC), are mediated by an array of cytokines, receptorsand adhesion molecules. The multiple myeloma microenvironment is formed by clonal plasma cells, extracellular proteins and BMSC, which are intimately involved in all biological stages of intramedullary tumor growth and angiogenesis (Fig. 1.6).

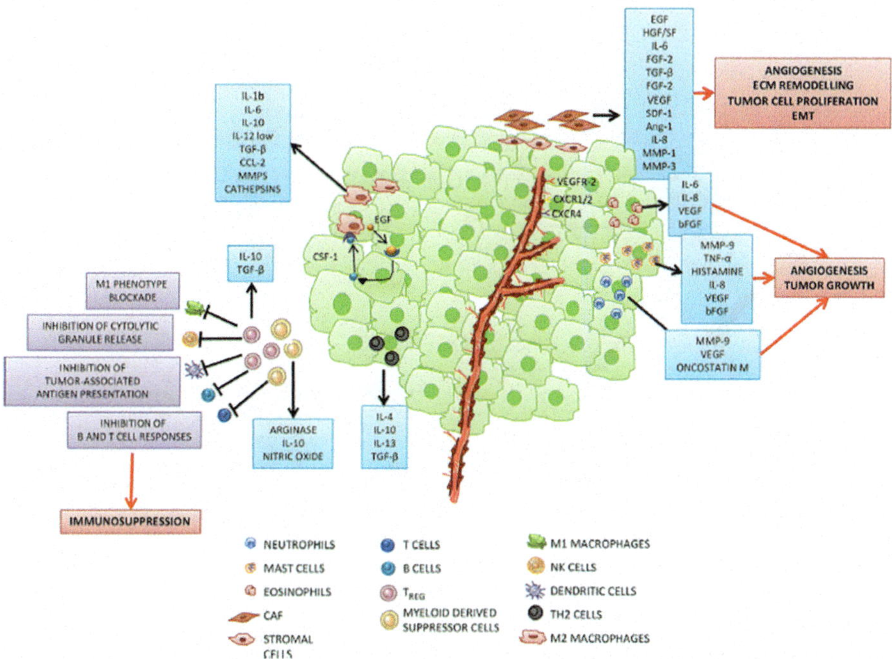

Fig. 1.4 Tumor microenvironment composed by tumor stroma, blood vessels and infiltrating inflammatory cells is characterized by a complex network of intercellular interactions between tumor and inflammatory cells. Different types of cells are found in the stroma, including fibroblasts, vascular smooth muscle, epithelial and immune cells. The latter cells comprise effectors of both adaptive immunity, such as T and B lymphocytes, and innate immunity, i.e. macrophages, dendritic cells (DCs), neutrophils, mast cells, eosinophils and natural killer (NK) cells. Most of the stromal cells participate in the promotion of the tumor growth. Cancer associated fibroblasts (CAFs) and M2 like polarized macrophages (tumor associated macrophages, TAMs), which can be induced by tumor-derived factors (for example, TGF-β, FGF or PDGF), support tumor growth, angiogenesis, extracellular matrix remodeling and epithelial mesenchymal transition (EMT), by secreting a plethora of pro-tumorigenic proteases, cytokines and growth factors. As tumors grow, immune-suppressor cells, including myeloid derived suppressor cells (MDSC) and T regulatory (T_{REG}) cells infiltrate the tumor to disrupt immune surveillance through multiple mechanisms, including inhibition of tumor-associated antigen presentation by DCs, T and B cell responses, NK cell cytotoxicity and blockade of M1 macrophage phenotype. Moreover, tumor progression is associated with the increase of TH2 cells secreting immunosuppressive molecules such as IL-4, IL-10 and TGF–β. Mast cells, neutrophils and eosinophils are also recruited to the tumor site where they secrete proliferative and pro-angiogenic factors (Reproduced from Raffaghello et al. 2014)

It is well established that tumor cells are able to secrete pro-angiogenic factors as well as mediators for inflammatory cells (Ribatti and Vacca 2008). They produce indeed angiogenic cytokines, which are exported from tumor cells or mobilized from the extracellular matrix. As a consequence, tumor cells are surrounded by an infiltrate of inflammatory cells. These cells communicate via a complex network of intercellular signaling pathways, mediated by surface adhesion molecules, cyto-

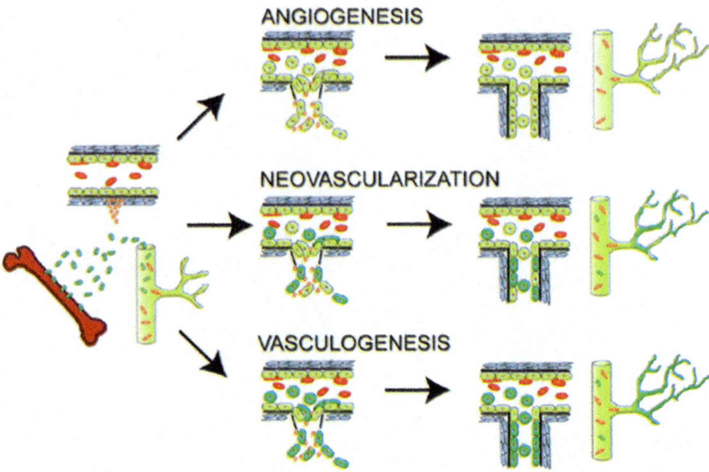

Fig. 1.5 Angiogenesis and vasculogenesis. During angiogenesis, pre-existing endothelial cells proliferate and migrate to form a new vessel. During vasculogenesis, a variety of factors induce mobilization of endothelial progenitor cells from the bone marrow into the peripheral circulation. Endothelial progenitor cells are recruited to the site of vascularization, differentiate, proliferate, migrate, and participate in vascular growth. (Reproduced from Afzal et al. 2007)

kines and their receptors (Ribatti et al. 2006b). Immune cells cooperate and synergize with stromal cells as well as malignant cells in stimulating endothelial cell proliferation and blood vessel formation. These synergies may represent important mechanisms for tumor development and metastasis by providing efficient vascular supply and easy pathway to escape. Indeed, the most aggressive human cancers are associated with a dramatic host response composed of various immune cells, especially macrophages and mast cells.

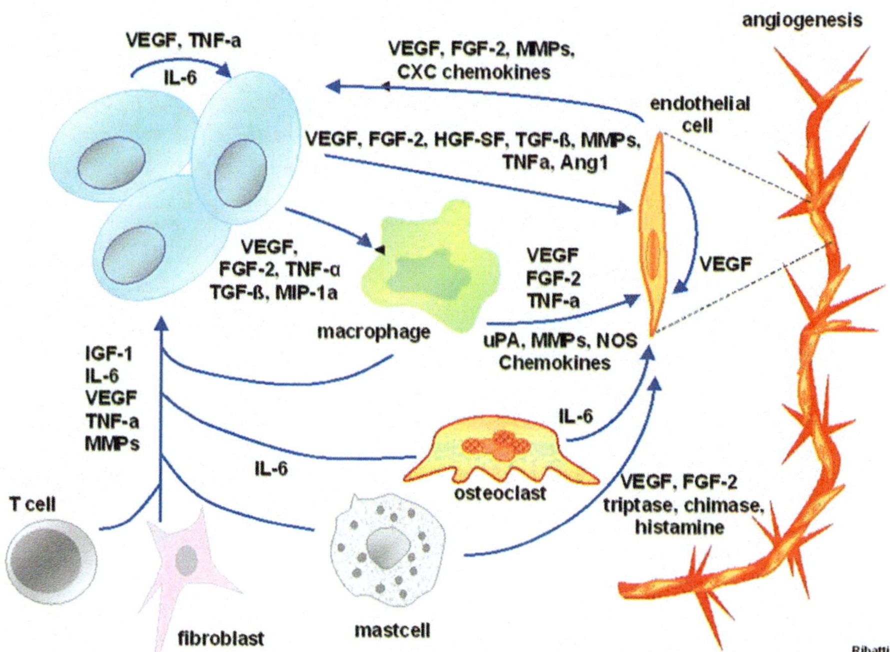

Fig. 1.6 Interplay between various microenvironmental cells and factors promoting angiogenesis in multiple myeloma (MM). The bone marrow contains hematopoietic stem cells (HSCs) and non-hematopoietic cells. HSCs are able to give rise to all types of mature blood cells, while the no hematopoietic component includes mesenchymal stem cells (MSCs), fibroblasts, osteoblasts, osteoclasts, chondroclasts, endothelial cells, endothelial progenitor cells, B and T lymphocytes, NK cells, erythrocytes, megakaryocytes, platelets, macrophages and mast cells. All of these cells form specialized "niches" in the bone marrow microenvironment which are close to the vasculature ("vascular niche") or to the endosteum ("osteoblast niche"). The "vascular niche" is rich in blood vessels where endothelial cells and mural cells (pericytes and smooth muscle cells) and create a microenvironment that affects the behavior of several stem and progenitor cells. The vessel wall serves as an independent niche for the recruitment of endothelial progenitor cells, MSCs and HSCs. The activation by angiogenic factors and inflammatory cytokines switch the "vascular niche" to promote MM tumor growth and spread (Reproduced from Ribatti et al. 2006b)

Chapter 2
The Importance of Microenvironment in Tumor Metastasis

In 1889, the English surgeon Stephen Paget (Fig. 2.1) published his "seed and soil" explanation of nonrandom pattern of metastasis, and was the first to suggest that interactions between tumor cells and host cells in the microenvironment are critical in regulating tumorigenesis (Paget 1889). Certain favored tumor cells (the 'seed'), he said, had a specific affinity for the growth-enhancing milieu within specific organs (the 'soil'), and hence metastasis only occurred when the 'seed' and 'soil' were compatible (Ribatti et al. 2006). Paget analyzed autopsy records of 735 women with breast cancer. His analysis documented a non-random pattern of metastasis to visceral organs and bones, suggesting that the process was not due to chance but rather that certain tumor cells had a specific affinity for the milieu of certain organs.

Auerbach (1988) in his comments about organ selectivity of metastasis writes: "Paget is almost apologetic as he contrasts the work of those that study the 'seed' to his own work on the 'soil': the best work in the pathology of cancer is done by those studying the nature of the 'seed'. They are like scientific botanists; and he who turns over the records of cases of cancer is only a ploughman, but his observations of the properties of the 'soil' may also be useful". Auerbach then adds: "Those individuals who study the properties of the host environment should not be ignored. Not only are the observations of the 'soil' useful, they provide essential information without which we will not be able to understand the nature of the metastatic process". Paget postulated that microenvironment provides a fertile 'soil' for cancer cells endowed with a capacity to grow under specific conditions provided by the 'soil'. A current definition of the 'seed and soil' hypothesis consists of three principles. First, neoplasms are biologically heterogeneous and contain subpopulations of cells with different angiogenic, invasive and metastatic properties. Second, the process of metastasis is selective for cells that succeed in invasion, embolization, survival in the circulation, arrest in a distant capillary bed, and extravasation into and moltiplication within the organ parenchyma. Third, the outcome of metastasis depends on multiple interactions of metastatic cells with homeostatic mechanisms, which the tumor cells can escape.

© Springer International Publishing AG 2017

D. Ribatti, *Inflammation and Angiogenesis*, https://doi.org/10.1007/978-3-319-68448-2_2

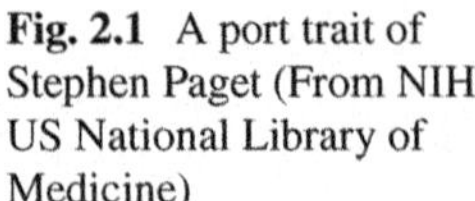

Fig. 2.1 A port trait of
Stephen Paget (From NIH
US National Library of
Medicine)

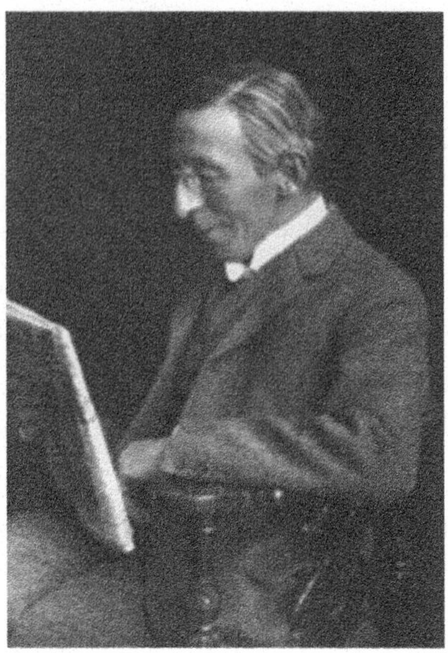

In 1989, in his introductory remarks to the symposium commemorating the anniversary of Paget's 'seed and soil' hypothesis, George Poste pointed out that: "There are few scientists, historically or contemporary, whose work will stand 100 years of scrutiny and not succumb to the depressing trend of modern publications – to ignore papers published more than five years ago".

The importance of several components of the 'soil' in regulating tumor growth has since been emphasized: (1) the extracellular matrix; (2) stromal cells and their growth factors and inhibitors; (3) microvessels and angiogenic factors and (4) inflammatory cells. It has long been accepted that most malignant tumors show an organ-specific pattern of metastasis. Colon carcinomas metastasize usually to liver and lung but rarely to bone, skin or brain and almost never to kidneys, intestine or muscle.

In contrast, other tumor entities, such as breast carcinomas, frequently form metastases in most of these organs. This specific formation of secondary tumors at distant sites appears to require a number of steps must be successfully completed by metastazing tumor cells (Chambers et al. 2002). Various explanations have been proposed for the site selectivity of blood-bone metastases, including tumor cell surface characteristics (Reading and Hutchins 1985), response to organ-derived chemotactic factors (Hujanen and Terranova 1985), adhesion between tumor cells and the target organ components (Nicolson 1988a, b) and response to specific host tissue growth factors (Nicolson and Dulski 1986). The relative importance of pre-existing tumor subpopulations with specific metastatic properties and the organ environment characteristics in determining metastatic homing have been debated (Fidler 1986; Nicolson 1988a; Talmadge and Fidler 1982; Weiss 1979).

An alternative explanation for the different sites of tumor growth involves interactions between the metastatic cells and the organ environment, possibly in terms of specific binding to endothelial cells and responses to local growth factors. Endothelial cells in the vasculature of different organs express different cell-surface receptors and growth factors that influence the phenotype of the corresponding metastases.

Greene and Harvey (1964) first suggested that the organ distribution patterns of metastatic foci were dependent on the formation of sufficient adhesive bonds between arrested tumor cells and endothelial cells, and they hypothesized that these interactions were similar to lymphocyte/endothelial cells at sites of inflammation. The development of organ-derived microvascular endothelial cell cultures has allowed more specific studies on the preferential homing of tumor cells.

Auerbach and co-workers (1985; 1987) found that different tumors showed differences in their adhesive propensity and preference for different endothelial cells, and in a few cases preferential adhesion was observed to the endothelial cells derived from the organ of origin and the target organ.

Chapter 3
Immune Cells

Immune cells can be divided into innate (myeloid) and adaptive (lymphoid) cells. Innate immune cells, including macrophages, polymorphonuclear granulocytes (neutrophils, basophils and eosinophils) mast cells, dendritic cells, natural killer cells and platelets represent the first line of defence against pathogens and foreign agents (Table 3.1).

Prior to the evolution of vertebrates, host defense against foreign invaders was mediated by the mechanisms of natural immunity, including phagocytic cells and circulating molecules that resemble component of the mammalian complement system. Whereas phagocytes and complement cannot distinguish between different antigens and are not specifically enhanced by repeated exposure to the same antigen, lymphocytes and antibodies are highly specific and their production or expansion is stimulated by foreign antigens.

The innate immune cells can directly eliminate pathogenic agents *in situ*. Dendritic cells, on the other hand, take up foreign antigens and migrate to lymphoid organs where they present their antigens to adpative immune cells. Adaptive immune cells are lymphocytes (T and B cells), which undergo clonal expansion and elaborate an adaptive response targeted to the foreign agent (Table 3.2). The activation of lymphocytes leads to the generation of numerous effector mechanisms, including the participation of mononuclear phagocytes and lymphocytes themselves. These cells are present in the blood, from where they can migrate to peripheral sites of antigen exposure and function to eliminate the antigen. The mediators of natural immunity include those that protect against viral infection and those that initiate inflammatory reactions that protect against bacteria (Table 3.3).

Whereas the cells of the innate immune system are found in the blood stream and in most organs of the body, lymphocytes are localized to specialized organs and tissues, where they interact with one another to initiate and amplify immune responses.

© Springer International Publishing AG 2017

D. Ribatti, *Inflammation and Angiogenesis*, https://doi.org/10.1007/978-3-319-68448-2_3

Table 3.1 Features of innate and acquired immunity

Natural
Physicochemical barriers (skin, mucous membranes)
Circulating molecules (complement)
Cells (neutrophils, macrophages, NK cells)
Soluble mediators (macrophage-derived cytokines)
Acquired
Physicochemical barriers (cutaneous and mucosal immune systems)
Circulating molecules (antibodies)
Cells (lymphocytes)
Soluble mediators (lymphocyte-derived cytokines)

Table 3.2 Lymphocytes classes

B lymphocytes
Function: Antibody production (humoral immunity)
T lymphocytes
Functions: stimuli for B cell growth and differentiation (helper); lysis of virus-infected cells, tumor cells and allografts (cytolitic); macrophage activation by secreted cytokines (cell-mediated immunity)
Natural killer cells
Functions: Lysis of virus-infected cells, tumor cells; antibody-dependent cellular cytotoxicity

Table 3.3 Principal mediators of natural immunity and of immune-mediated inflammation

Natural immunity
Interferon alpha and beta
Tumor necrosis factor, the principal mediator of the host response to gram-negative bacteria
Interleukin-1
Interleukin-6, serves as a growth factor for activated B lymphocytes in the sequence of their differentiation
Chemokines, a large family of structurally homologous cytokines, approximately 8–10 kD in size
Immune mediated inflammation
Interferon gamma, a potent acitivator of mononuclear phagocytes
Lymphotoxin
Interleukin-5
Interleukin-10
Interleukin-12, the most potent NK cell stimulator
Migration inhibitory factor

Chapter 4
Lymphocyte Homing

There is tight interplay between innate immune cells and the vascular system. Endothelial cells mediate immune cell recruitment to extravascular tissues by expressing a repertoire of leukocyte adhesion molecules. TNF-α and IL-1 increase the expression of E-selectin and vascular adhesion molecule-1 (V-CAM-1) on endothelial cells, promoting leukocyte adhesion and homing to sites of inflammation (Balkwill 2002). The attachment of lymphocytes to the endothelium is mediated by several homing receptors and other cell adhesion molecules on the lymphocytes and their corresponfing ligands on endothelial cells (Table 4.1).

The sequence of events in the extravasation of leukocytes from the vascular lumen to the extracellular space include margination and rolling, adhesion and transmigration between endothelial cells, and migration in interstitial tissues toward a chemotactic stimulus. Neutrophils, monocytes, eosinophils, and lymphocytes use different molecules for rolling and adhesion.

The best characterized lymphocyte homing receptors is L-selectin, the molecule that mediates the binding of naïve lymphocytes to post-capillary high endothelial venules (HEVs) found in the inner cortex of peripheral lymph nodes and thymus. HEVs are specialized venules lined by plump endothelial cells that protrude into the vessel lumen. HEVs are also present in mucosal lymphoid tissues, such as Peyer's patches in the gut, in the internodular lymphatic tissue of tonsils, appendix, but not in the spleen. When T lymphocytes collide with the endothelium lining an HEV they remain loosely attached for several seconds, while normally lymphocytes coursing through the microcirculation randomly collide with vessel walls and either immediately rebound or adhere to the lining endothelial cells for only a fraction of a second before they are dislodged by the shear force of flowing blood. The unsusual height of the endothelium is explained as a special adaptation reducing to a minimum loss of fluid, when lymphocytes migrate from blood to lymphatic tissue.

Vascular endothelial cells, in response to TNFα and other cytokines, produce vasodilators that increase leukocyte delivery to tissues; express adhesion molecules including E-selectin, V-CAM-1 and I-CAM-1, that bind leukocytes; synthesize and express chemokines that activate leukocytes, increasing integrin affinity and cell

© Springer International Publishing AG 2017

D. Ribatti, *Inflammation and Angiogenesis*, https://doi.org/10.1007/978-3-319-68448-2_4

Table 4.1 Lymphocyte
homing receptors

Homing of naïve T lymphocytes in peripheral lymph nodes
T cell homing receptor (L-selectin, LFA-1)
Endothelia ligand (GlyCAM1)
Homing of T cells to mucosal tissues (e.g., Peyer's patches)
T cell homing receptor ($\alpha4\beta7$ integrin;CD44)
Endothelial ligand (Mad CAM-1)
Homing of memory and effector T cells to peripheral tissues
T cell homing receptor (VLA-4; LFA-1; CD44)
Endothelial ligand (V-CAM-1; ICAM-1, −2; Hyaluronate)

motility; allow plasma proteins (fibrinogen and fibronectin) to leak into the tissues, forming a scaffold for leukocytes.

On the other hand, innate immune cells synthesize a number of soluble factors that influence endothelial cell behavior. In addition, many of the mediators that are involved in angiogenesis, are also inflammatory molecules. Recruitment of an inflammatory infiltrate supports angiogenesis and tissue remodeling.

Lymphocyte recirculation through the blood takes about 0.6 hour, transit through the spleen requires about 6 hours, and passage through lymph nodes 15–20 hours. During the period of recirculation, lymphocytes do not divide. The purpose of lymphocyte recirculation is to anable immunocompetent lymphocytes to inform lymphopoietic organs about the presence or absence of antigens in the body.

Chapter 5
Inflammation and Cancer

The association between inflammation and cancer was discovered as early as 1863 by Rudolf Virchow (Fig. 5.1) (Virchow 1863), who first described the presence of a leukocyte infiltrate in tumor tissues (Balkwill and Mantovani 2001). Individuals affected by chronic inflammatory pathologies have increased risk of cancer development, since they lead to the release of proinflammatory cytokines, creating a favourable microenvironment for tumor progression and metastasis (Balkwill et al. 2005). Examples include viral infection with hepatitis B and C for liver cancer; papilloma virus for cervix carcinoma; bacterial infections, such as *Helicobacter pylori* for gastric cancer or lymphoma; parasites, such as Schistosoma for bladder cancer. It is thought that *Helicobacter pylori* infection leads to the formation of *Helicobacter pylori* reactive T cells, which in turn cause polyclonal B-cell proliferation. In some patients viral integrations causes secondary rearrangements of chromosomes, including multiple deletions that may harbor unknown suppressor genes.

Epidemiologic data indicate that over 25% of cancers are related to chronic inflammation (Hussain and Harris 2007; Vendramini-Costa and Carvalho 2012).

The inflammation generates oxidative stress which in tunr generates reactive oxygen spescies (ROS), that cause DNA damage and chromosomal instability and by enhancing tumor cell proliferation and resistance to apoptosis. Cytokines, chemokines, free radicals, prostaglandins, enzymes, and matrix metalloproteinases released by inflammatory cells can induce genetic and epigenetic changes that can lead to development and progression of cancer. During chronic inflammation, a wide array of intracellular signaling pathways, including cell surface receptors, kinases, and transcription factors, are often dysregulated, leading to abnormal expression of pro-inflammatory genes involved in malignant transformation (Vendramini-Costa and Carvalho 2012). Among these, STAT3 has emerged as a critical regulator of tumor-associated inflammation. Targeting STAT3 has the potential to not only inhibit tumor growth directly, but also to alter the immunological environment so as to favor control of tumor proliferation. Cytokines and growth factors can also upregulate the expression and enhance the activity of NOX family members in epithelial cells, increasing ROS production in the tumor

© Springer International Publishing AG 2017

D. Ribatti, *Inflammation and Angiogenesis*, https://doi.org/10.1007/978-3-319-68448-2_5

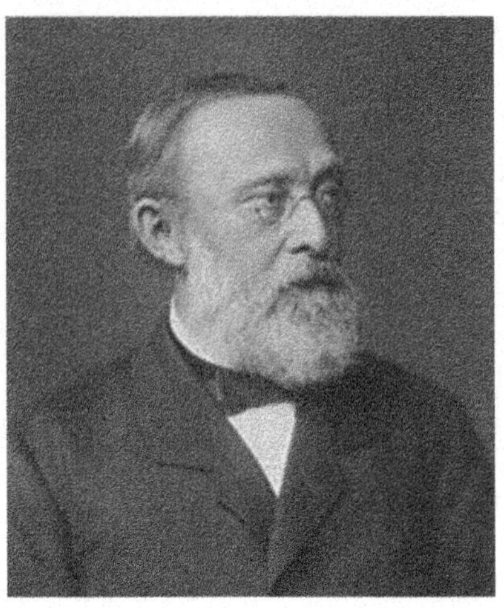

microenvironment, which damages genomic DNA and may produce mutational hits that can initiate tumor formation. In this context, the ROS scavenger NAC slows tumor progression in a p53-dependent mouse lymphomagenesis model by reducing ROS-mediated genomic instability (Sablina et al. 2005), and the NOX inhibitors decrease the growth of human colon cancer xenografts in vivo (Doroshow et al. 2013).

Leukocytes that do reach the tumor often remain localized in the tumor periphery or stroma and are often not able to exert strong antitumor activity. Both innate and adaptive immune cells are capable of polarization into their "tumoricidal" (growth arresting) or "tumorigenic" (growth promoting) forms that influence the growth, proliferation and infiltration of other immune cells at the site of injury by expression of appropriate signals/mediators. In some cancers, inflammation precede development of malignancy, and it is well known that tumor-infiltrated inflammatory cells produce various cytokines that regulate the inflammatory response in tumor-bearing hosts, while inflammatory cells may produce growth factors that suppress antitumor immune response. In neoplastic tissues, inflammatory cells act in concert with tumor cells, stromal cells and endothelial cells to create a microenvironment that is critical for the survival, development and dissemination of the neoplastic mass (Hanahan and Weinberg 2011). These interactions within the tumor microenvironment may represent important mechanisms for tumor development and metastasis by providing an efficient vascular supply and an easy escape pathway. Among inflammatory cells that have been identified as modifiers of tumor microenvironment, mast cells and macrophages play a crucial role.

Micro RNAs (miRNAs) are involved in many types of inflammatory responses. The miRNA miR-21. miR-125, and miR-155 are the most frequently expressed during infection and may have a potential role in carcinogenesis induced by infection agents (O'Connell et al. 2012; Iliopoulos 2014).

5.1   The Relationship Between the Immune System Surveillance and Cancer

In 1909, Paul Ehrlich (Fig. 5.2) formulated the hypothesis that host defense may prevent neoplastic cells from developing into tumors (Ehrlich 1909). He stated that: "In the enormously complicated course of fetal and post-fetal development, aberrant cells become unusually common. Fortunately, in the majority of people, they remain completely latent thanks to the organism's positive mechanisms." (Ehrlich 1909). This hypothesis was not proven experimentally at the time due to the inadequacy of experimental tools and knowledge. The historical observations by Ehrlich that tumor cells are recognized and eliminated by the immune cells evolved in the theory of immune surveillance (Ribatti 2017).

Later, some biologists suggest the existence of an "immunological surveillance mechanism" against tumor cells. Lewis Thomas suggested that the immune system recognize newly arising tumors through the expression of tumor specific neo-antigens and to eliminate them, similarly to homograft rejection, maintaining tissue homeostasis in complex multicellular organism (Thomas 1957). The first clear demonstration of specific capability to stimulate an immune response was made by Gross in 1953 after intradermal immunization of C3H mice, obtained by continuous brother to sister mating for more 20 years, against a sarcoma (Gross 1943), followed by Foley in 1953 in methylcholantrene-induced tumors (Foley 1953).

Sir Frank Mac Farlane Burnet (Fig. 5.3) hypothesized that tumor cell neo-antigens induce an immunological reaction against cancer and subsequently formulated the immune surveillance theory (Burnet 1957, 1970). He wrote that: "It is by no means inconceivable that small accumulation of tumor cells may develop and because of their

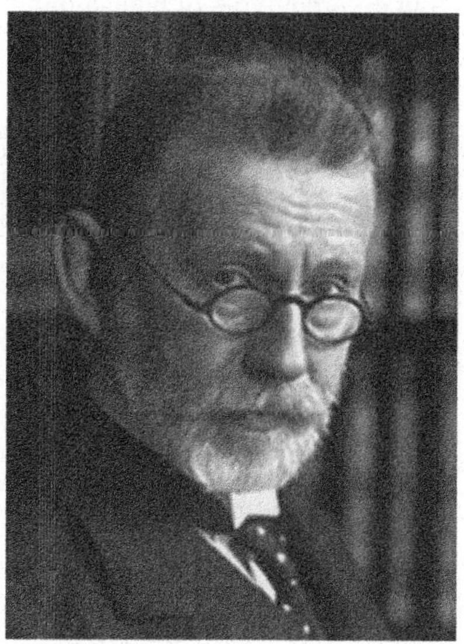

Fig. 5.2 A port trait of Paul Ehrlich (from Nobel Prize Organization)

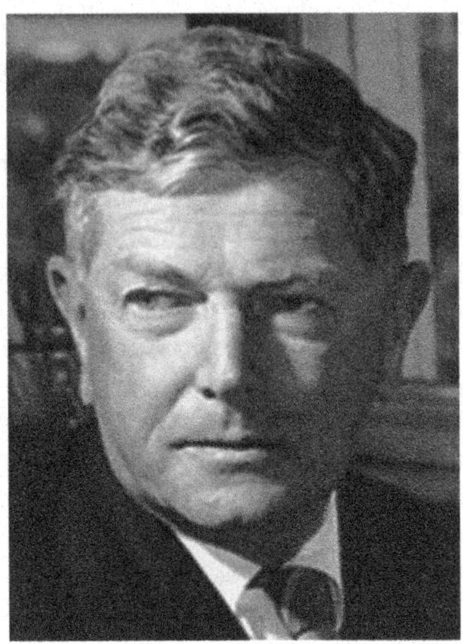

Fig. 5.3 A port trait of Sir Frank Macfarlane Burnet (from Nobel Prize Organization)

possession of new antigenic potentialities provoke an effective immunological reaction with regression of the tumor and no clinical hint of its existence." (Burnet 1970).

In transplantation models, tumors are rejected in syngeneic hosts, while transplantation of normal tissues are accepted, confirming the existence of tumor-specific antigens (Table 5.1) (Burnet 1970). Professional antigen presenting cells process and present tumor associated antigens (via cross presentation of debris, perhaps due to spontaneous tumor cell lysis, or perhaps due to NK cell destruction, or other processes such as "nibbling") to immune cells, and generate memory and effector cells which survey the body, seeking out tumor cells.

In different types of human tumors, including melanoma, cancer of breast, bladder, colon, prostate, ovary, rectum, and for glioblastoma (Clemente et al. 1996; Rilke et al. 1991; Nacopoulou et al. 1981; Epstein and Fatti 1976; Deligdisch et al. 1982; Jass 1986; Palma et al. 1978), a longer survival has been observed in patients with a higher number of lymphocytes and NK cells. These latter do not require prior sensitization for efficient tumor cell lysis and following activation with interleukin-2 (IL-2), NK cells can kill tumor cells (Waldhauer and Steinle 2008). Regulatory T cells (Tregs) exert both detrimental and beneficial effects to the host (Nishikawa and Sakaguchi 2010; Facciabene et al. 2012). Tumor antigens can be recognized by T cells, in cooperation with major histocompatibility complex (MHC) allowing T cells to interact with the antigen presenting cells (Boon and van der Bruggen 1996).

Athymic nude mice, traditionally considered to lack T cells, did not develop significantly more spontaneous or methylcholantrene-induced tumors than control mice (Stutman 1974; Outzen et al. 1975). In this experimental condition, the immune response mediated by T and NK cells was similar in immunocompetent and nude mice. IFNγ and perforin, are both involved in prevent tumor formation in

Table 5.1 Different class of tumor antigens

| **Cancer-testis antigens** |
| Encoded by genes that are silent in all adult tissues except the testis. Prototypic of this group is the MAGE family of genes |
| **Tissue specific antigens** |
| MART-1, gp100 |
| **Antigens resulting from mutational changes in proteins** |
| Products of βcatenin, RAS, TP53, CDK4 genes |
| **Overexpressed antigens** |
| HER-2 |
| **Viral antigens** |
| Antigens derived from oncogenic viruses such as HPV and EBV |
| **Oncofetal antigens** |
| Carcinoembryonic antigen (CEA) and α-fetoprotein (AFP). |
| Increased levels of CEA can be found in association with neoplasms of different histogenesis and may also occur in association with some non-neoplastic conditions. AFP may appear in the plasma of up to 50% patients with malignant germ cell tumors. |
| **Differentiation-specfic antigens** |
| CD10 and prostate-specific antigen (PSA) |
| **Other tumor antigens** |
| MUC-1 antigen |

mice (Kaplan et al. 1998; Shankaran et al. 2001). In fact, neutralization of IFNγ resulted in rapid growth of tumors (Dighe et al. 1994), and mice lacking IFNγ were more sensitive to methylcholantherene-induced carcinogenesis (Kaplan et al. 1998). However, treatment with IFNγ had no benefit for patients with different type of tumors (Gleave et al. 1998; Wiesenfeld et al. 1995; Jett et al. 1994). Perforin inhibited B cell lymphoma development (van den Broek et al. 1996; Bolitho et al. 2009; Street et al. 2004). Moreover, mutations in the gene encoding perforin have been demonstrated in lymphoma patients (Clementi et al. 2005).

Individuals with primary or secondary immunodeficiences and therapy to prevent transplant rejection are associated with a higher incidence of cancer (Melief and Schwartz 1975). About 5% of individual with congenital immunodeficiencies develop cancers, a rate that is about 200 times thst for individuals without such immunodeficiences. Cancers most commonly found in immunodeficient individuals are virus-associated (Schulz 2009), including Epstein-Barr virus-related tumors (Gaidano and Dalla-Favera 1992; Ru-Chen 2011). Failure of human herpes virus (HHV) immune response is one of the factors involved in the pathogenesis of Kaposi sarcoma (Mesri et al. 1996). Several other cancers, have increased incidences in persons with human immunodeficiency virus (HIV)/AIDS, including hepatocellular carcinoma, which is frequently associated with infection with the hepatitis B or C virus (Mesri et al. 1996). Merkel cell carcinoma, a rare skin cancer that occurs more frequently after organ transplantation or B-cell malignancy, conditions of suppressed or disordered immunity, has an increased incidence in HIV-infected individuals (Engels et al. 2002). Associations between different bacteria, including *Helicobacter pylori* and clamyidia, and higher incidence of various tumors have been described (Mc Farlane and Munro 1997; Silva et al. 2014). Bacteria are capable of homing to tumors when systemically administered, resulting in high levels of replication locally (Morrissey et al. 2010; Toso et al. 2002). However, the frequency of non-virally induced tumors, is not increased among transplant recipients (Chapman et al. 2013). Immune competence decreases with age, the so-called "immunosenescence", implying that decreased immunosurveillance against cancer contribute to increased disease in the elderly (Pawelec et al. 2010). Cytomegalovirus (CMV) and EBV infection are determinants of immunosenescence (Fulop et al. 2010).

Immunosuppression may be not associated to an increase of tumors (Martinez 1964; Penn 1988). In fact, thymectomy at birth reduced the incidence of mammary adenocarcinoma (Yunis et al. 1969), and immunologic reconstitution restored the susceptibility to tumor (Penn 1988). The incidence of mammary carcinomas decreases in immunosuppressed individuals (Stewart et al. 1995). Finally, leprosy and sarcoidosis which are characterized by immunosuppression, are not associated to an increased incidence of tumors (Stutman 1975).

5.2 Immunoediting, a New Approach

As Sirvastava (2006) said: "The immune surveillance hypothesis is often regarded as the intellectual underpinning of cancer immunology. Although the hypothesis itself has contributed little to our attempts to treat cancer through immunological means, it has profound implications for understanding the functions of the immune system." Dunn and Schreiber developed the concept of "cancer immunoediting" (Fig. 5.4), composed of three phases (Dunn et al. 2002). In the first one, the elimination phase, tumor cells are killed by NK, CD4$^+$ and CD8$^+$ cells (Gasser and Raulet 2006). The second phase corresponds to a state of equilibrium between immune and tumor cells. When the immune system is unable to destroy the tumor, the third phase, corresponding to the escape phase, develops which concludes with the appearance of clinically detectable tumors.

Multiple myeloma progresses from the monoclonal gammopathy of undetermined significance (MGUS) to asymptomatic and, respectively, symptomatic myeloma (Dhodapkar 2005). In this context, it is possible demonstrate that T cells from patients with MGUS develop an immune reaction to premalignant cells, which instead is absent in patients with multiple myeloma and the transition to multiple myeloma correspond to tumor escape phase (Dhodapkar et al. 2003).

The escape phase is characterized by the selection of tumor variants which will progress later on (Corthay 2014; Teng et al. 2015; Muenst et al. 2016); by a down-regulation or loss of the expression of tumor antigens; by an upregulation of resistance against tumor cells and/or an increased expression of pro-survival genes, and finally by the development of an immunosuppressive tumor microenvironment (Dunn et al. 2004). Moreover, the establishment of a condition of

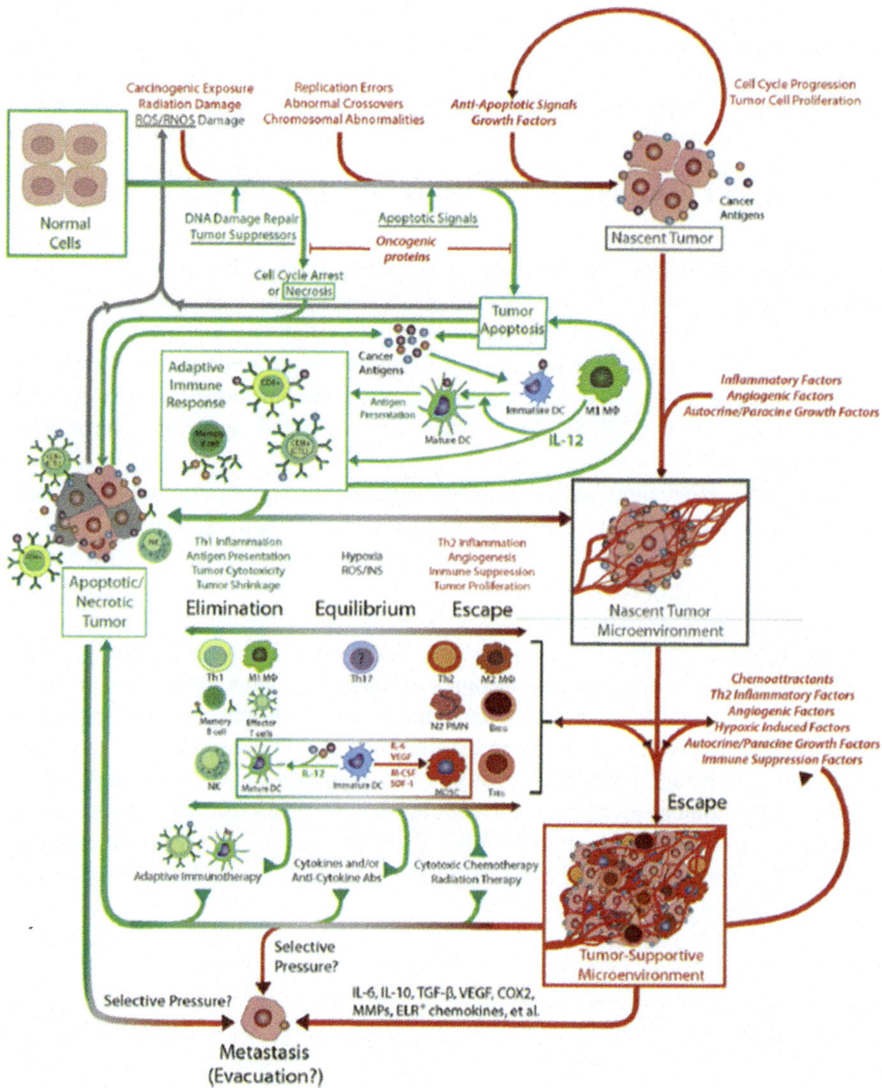

Fig. 5.4 A model of immunoediting in tumor progression. Normal cells may become nascent tumors by evading tumor suppression after carcinogenic mutation and/or apoptosis that would normally result from gross chromosomal changes. Pro-inflammatory and pro-angiogenic factors can help to establish blood supply for the growing nascent tumor. Activation of the adaptive or native immune response can eliminate the nascent tumor, the tumor may remain in equilibrium as an occult tumor, or the tumor may escape immunosurveillance to create a viable tumor-supportive microenvironment. Innate and adaptive immune responses may still work to eliminate the tumor via immunosurveillance. Tumors may also metastasize to move to another location; this may be an additional mechanism of avoiding immunosurveillance. Green color denotes processes potentially leading to tumor eradication, while red color means promoting tumor escape and progression (Reproduced from Burkholder et al. 2014)

central and peripheral immune tolerance, involving the activation of Tregs is crucial for the establishment of an escape mechanism (Dunn et al. 2004; Schwann and Smyth 2007).

5.3   Current Approaches in Anti-tumor Immunotherapy

Some analysts have predicted that within 10 years, immunotherapy will constitute 60% of all cancer treatments (Ledford 2014). A novel group of immunomodulatory antibodies has been introduced in the clinical use, which can break tumor specific immune tolerance and induce regression of tumors. These antibodies block growth signals of tumor cells, or induce apoptosis. Since the introduction of rituximab (Cheson and Leonard 2008), 13 further tumor-directed antibodies have been approved.

Three of the most significant therapeutic approaches are represented by sipuleu-cel-T, an immunotherapeutic vaccine for prostate cancer (Gulley et al. 2015); ipili-mumab, a check point inhibitor of CTLA-4, and anti-programmed death receptor-1 (PD-1) and its ligand PDL-1 antibodies (anti-PD-1/PD-L-1) (He et al. 2004; Blank et al. 2004; Philips and Atkins 2015) for the treatment of metastatic melanoma.

Currently, cancer immunotherapies are classified as active and passive treatments. Active treatments include vaccines designed to induce tumor cell recognition. Passive treatments, on the other hand, imply direct administration of antibodies and T cells, to the patient. In this context, immune checkpoint inhibitors and adoptive T cell therapy are among the most innovative approaches (Sharma and Allison 2015). At the clinical level, it is not yet clarified why certain patients respond to specific types of immunotherapies, while others do not. The development of future treatments depends on finding effective immune-based biomarkers that can help to predict responses to treatment.

Chapter 6
Inflammation and Angiogenesis

There is increasing evidence to support the view that angiogenesis and inflammation are mutually dependent (Fig. 6.1) (Mueller 2008). During inflammatory reactions, immune cells synthesize and secrete pro-angiogenic factors that promote neovascularization. Among the cytokines, IL-6, TNF-α and CXCR2 chemokine receptor and its ligand promote angiogenesis in tumor microenvironment.

On the other hand, the newly formed vascular supply contributes to the perpetuation of inflammation by promoting the migration of inflammatory cells to the site of inflammation (Mueller 2008). The extracellular matrix and basement membrane are a source for endogenous angiogenesis inhibitors activated through the action of matrix metalloproteinases. On the other hand, many extracellular matrix molecules promote angiogenesis by stabilizing blood vessels and sequestering angiogenic molecules (Nyberg et al. 2008).

It is well established that tumor cells are able to secrete pro-angiogenic factors as well as mediators for inflammatory cells (Ribatti and Vacca 2008). They produce indeed angiogenic cytokines, which are exported from tumor cells or mobilized from the extracellular matrix. As a consequence, tumor cells are surrounded by an infiltrate of inflammatory cells. Immune cells cooperate and synergise with stromal cells as well as malignant cells in stimulating endothelial cell proliferation and blood vessel formation. These synergies may represent important mechanisms for tumor development and metastasis by providing efficient vascular supply and easy pathway to escape. Indeed, the most aggressive human cancers are associated with a dramatic host response composed of various immune cells, especially macrophages and mast cells (Mueller 2008).

Inflammation-associated angiogenesis also occurs during pathophysiological reactions, like wound healing and scar formation. The process of extracellular matrix remodeling that accompanies this kind of tissue responses is strictly dependent upon angiogenic events. Inflammatory cells contribute even to angiogenesis concomitant with physiological processes, such as ovulation and endometrial vascularization during the reconstructive phase of the menstrual cycle and in pregnancy.

© Springer International Publishing AG 2017

D. Ribatti, *Inflammation and Angiogenesis*, https://doi.org/10.1007/978-3-319-68448-2_6

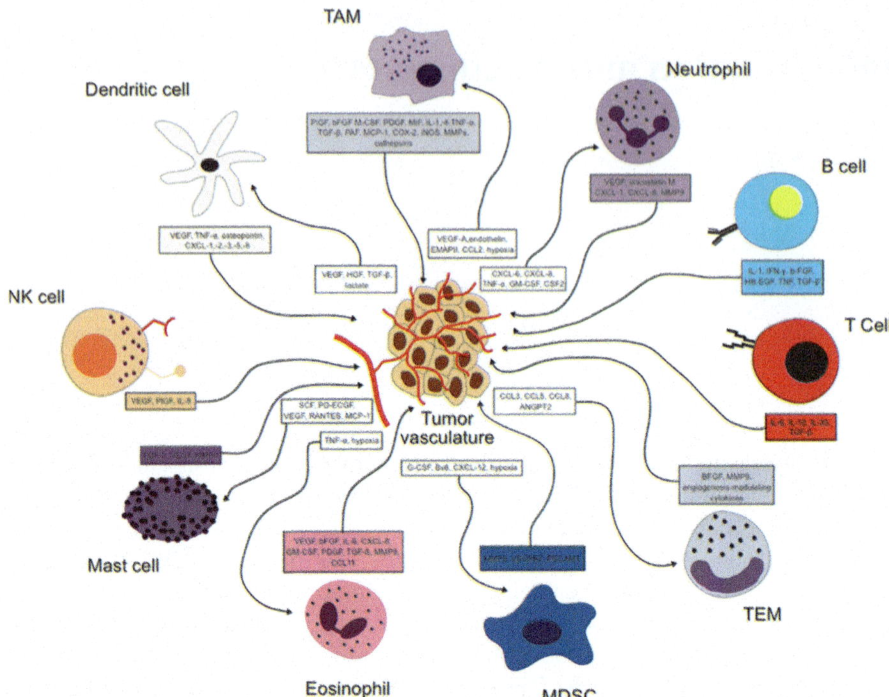

Fig. 6.1 Reciprocal interactions between different immune cell types and the tumor vasculature in the tumor microenvironment (Reproduced from Stockmann et al. 2014)

There is increasing evidence to support the view that angiogenesis is an integral component of a diverse range of chronic inflammatory and autoimmune diseases, including atherosclerosis, rheumatoid arthritis, diabetic retinopathy, psoriasis, airway inflammation, peptic ulcers, and Alzheimer's disease. Indeed, angiogenesis is intrinsic to chronic inflammation and is associated with structural changes, including activation and proliferation of endothelial cells, capillary and venule remodeling, all of which result in expansion of the tissue microvascular bed. Chronic inflammation in the airways, for instance, is associated with dramatic architectural changes in the walls of the airways and in the vasculature they contain. Therefore, it seems that an imbalance in favour of pro-angiogenic factors leads to the abnormal growth of new blood vessels in asthma. Inflammatory diseases, such as rheumatoid arthritis and psoriasis, are characterized by proliferating tissue containing an abundance of inflammatory cells and newly formed blood vessels. During prolonged inflammatory reactions, many structural and resident cells, such as fibroblasts, epithelial cells, smooth muscle cells, mast cells, and/or infiltrating cells, such as monocytes/macrophages, neutrophils, lymphocytes and eosinophils, synthesize and secrete pro-angiogenic factors that promote neovascularization. The anatomic expansion of the microvascular bed combined with its increased functional activation can therefore foster further recruitment of inflammatory cells, and angiogenesis and inflammation become chronically codependent processes.

Chapter 7
The Contribution of Immune Cells to Angiogenesis in Inflammation and Tumor Growth

7.1 Neutrophils

Neutrophils represent the most abundant leukocyte subpopulation in human peripheral blood and play an important role in host defence against pathogens during the earliest phases of inflammatory processes. Neutrophils are considered as macrophages, i.e. capable to phagocyte small particles such as bacteria, viruses, and small pieces of cell debris. Similarly to tumor associated macrophages (TAMs), tumor associated neutrophils (TANs) can exert both anti-tumoral and pro-tumoral functions (Fig. 7.1) (Fridlender et al. 2009).

A characteristic of neutrophils is the abundance of cytoplasmic granules. Mature neutrophils contain several types of granules and the diversity of granules appears to be linked to the timing of biosynthesis during myelopoiesis. The azurophilic or primary granules are formed during promyelocytic stage, are considered as primary lysosomes, and contain many antimicrobial compounds (Table 7.1). Specific or secondary granules are formed later, in the myelocyte, and are released in the extracellular space (Table 7.2). When the peroxidase reaction was introduced, the azurophilic granules were found to be peroxidase-positive as a result of the presence of the major myeloid protein, myeloperoxidase (MPO), and the specific granules were named peroxidase-negative granules. Gelatinase or tertiary granules were initially identified as gelatinase-containing granules and also contain many membrane proteins that are up-regulated to the cell surface after stimulation. Secretory vesicles distributed in the plasma membrane fraction have also described (Table 7.3).

Granulocyte-Colony Stimulating Factor (G-CSF), Granulocyte-Macrophage Colony Stimulating Factor (GM-CSF) and IL-10 activate signal transducer and activator of transcription (STAT) in neutrophils. Production of IL-8 has been extensively studied in neutrophils (Cheng and Kunkel 2003). Some of the stimuli that induced the expression of IL-8, induce the production of other pro-inflammatory agents, including growth-related oncogene (GRO)-α, TNFα IL-1β, oncostatin M, and C-C chemokines. In addition, neutrophils produce other anti-inflammatory agents, including

© Springer International Publishing AG 2017

D. Ribatti, *Inflammation and Angiogenesis*, https://doi.org/10.1007/978-3-319-68448-2_7

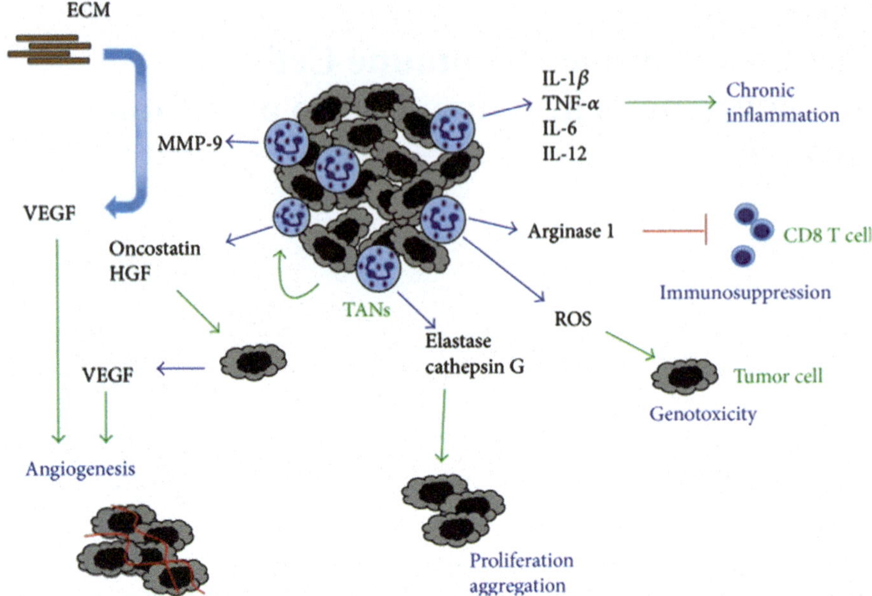

Fig. 7.1 Tumor-associated neutrophils (TANs) help tumor progression in several ways. TANs can secrete matrix metalloproteinase-9 (MMP-9) that releases vascular endothelial growth factor (VEGF) from the extracellular matrix (ECM) to promote angiogenesis. TAN can secrete cytokines (IL-1β, TNF-α, IL-6, and IL-12) that induce a chronic inflammatory state and arginase 1, which inhibits CD8 T cells, creating an immunosuppressive state. TANs also produce reactive oxygen species (ROS) that can damage DNA, inducing genotoxic effects on tumor cells. Serine proteases, such as elastase and cathepsin G, from neutrophil granules induce tumor cell proliferation. Certain tumors, like breast cancer cells, induce neutrophils to produce oncostatin, an IL-6-like cytokine that then stimulates breast cancer cells to secrete VEGF to promote angiogenesis (red lines represent new blood vessels). Also, hepatocellular carcinoma cells induce neutrophils to release hepatocyte growth factor (HGF), which activates tumor cells to become more invasive. Blue arrows denote molecules secreted by cells. Green arrows denote the action of molecules on cells (Reproduced from Uribe-Querol and Rosales 2015)

IL-1 receptor antagonist (IL-1RA) and TGF-β. Moreover, neutrophils are capable of phenotypic changes depending on the tissue microenvironment.

Some of neutrophils are free in the circulation, while others roll along the endothelium of small vessels. Duirng inflammation, much of the sequestration and infiltration occurs through vessels. The migration of neutrophils from blood into tissues involves a series of sequential adhesive steps, starting from the rolling adhesion on endothelium in postcapillary venules (Ley et al. 2007).

Neutrophilia occurs with many acute bacterial infections. It occurs less predictably with infections caused by viruses, fungi, and parasites. Chronic inflammatory diseases, including dermatitis, bronchitis, rheumatoid arthritis, osteomyelitis, ulcerative colitis, and gout, may cause a persistent neutrophilia. Recruitment of neutrophils to tumors is in part mediated by CXCL chemokines through the cognate receptors CXCR1 and CXCR2 (Coffelt et al. 2016). Moreover, neutrophilia is asso-

Table 7.1 Content of neutrophil azurophil (primary) granules

Membrane
CD 63, CD66c, CD68
Matrix
Lysozime
Difensins
Elastase
Cathepsin B, D, G
Proteinase 3
Esterase N
Alpha1-antitrypsin
Alpha-mannosidase
Azurocidin
Bacterial permeability-increasing protein
Beta-glycerolphosphatase
Beta-glucoronidase
Beta-galactosidase
Beta-glucosaminidase
Alpha-fucosidase
Acid mucopolysaccharidase
N-acethyl-beta-glocosaminidase
Sialidase
Ubiquiptin protein

ciated with lung and gastrointestinal malignancies, particularly when they metastasize to the liver and lung.

Evidence for the possible role of polymorphonuclear granulocytes in inflammation-mediated angiogenesis and tissue remodeling was initially provided by the finding that CXC receptor-2 (CXCR-2)-deficient mice, which lack neutrophil infiltration in thioglycollate-induced peritonitis (Cacalano et al. 1994), showed delayed angiogenesis and impaired cutaneous wound healing (Devalaraja et al. 2000).

Neutrophils are a source of soluble mediators which exert important angiogenic and anti-angiogenic functions. VEGF, IL-8, TNF-α, HGF and MMPs are the most important activators of angiogenesis produced by these cells (Dubravec et al. 1990; Bazzoni et al. 1991; Grenier et al. 2002). In this perspective, microarray analysis has revealed about 30 angiogenesis-relevant genes in human polymorphonuclear granulocytes (Schruefer et al. 2006). Thus, neutrophil contribute to tumor angiogenesis in several cancers (colorectal carcinoma, hepatocellular carcinoma, melanoma, squamous cell carcinoma, non small cell lung carcinoma, bronchoalveolar adenoarcinoma, non Hodgkin's lymphoma, and gastric carcinoma). Angiogenesis may be sustained by an autocrine amplification mechanism that allows persistent VEGF release to occur at sites of neutrophil accumulation. Production and release of VEGF from neutrophils depends from G-CSF (Ohki

Table 7.2 Content of neutrophil specific (secondary) granules

Membrane
CD11b, CD15, CD 66a, CD 66b
Cytocrome B558
FMLP receptor
Fibronectin receptor
G-protein alpha-subunit
Laminin receptor
NB1 antigen
Rap1, Rap2
Thrombospondin receptor
Tumor necrosis factor receptor
Vitronectin receptor
Matrix
Apolactofettin
Lyszoime
Beta2-microglobulin
Collagenase
Gelatinase
Histaminase
Heparanase
Pro-u-PA
Vitamin B12-binding protein
Sialidase
Protein kinase C inhibitor
SGP 28

Table 7.3 Content of neutrophil secretory vesicles

Membrane
CD10, CD13, CD16, CD35, CD45
Alkaline phosphatase
u-PA receptor
DAF
Matrix
Plasma proteins (including tetranectin and albumin)
Pro-u-PA
uPA

et al. 2005), and neutrophil-derived VEGF stimulates neutrophil migration (Ancelin et al. 2004). Neutrophils induce the sprouting of capillary-like structures in *in vitro* angiogenesis assay, mediated by secretion of both preformed VEGF (Mc Court et al. 1999) from cell stores and *de novo* synthesized IL-8.

Bv8 (also known as prokinecitin-2) promotes neutrophil mobilization and angiogenesis. In a tumor xenograft model, G-CSF induced the expression of Bv8 in neutrophils and blocking Bv8 impaired neutrophil recruitment, tumor growth, and angiogenesis (Shojaei et al. 2007, 2008). Neutrophils produce Bv8 that in turn can promote further neutrophil recruitment and directly stimulate vascular remodeling (Shojaei et al. 2008). Tumors resistant to anti-VEGF therapy displayed high neutrophil infiltration and resistance was due to G-CSF-induced Bv8 expression (Shojaei et al. 2009).

In breast cancer, release by tumor-associated and tumor-infiltrating neutrophils of oncostatin M, promotes tumor progression by enhancing angiogenesis and metastases (Queen et al. 2005). In addition, neutrophil-derived oncostatin M induces VEGF production from cancer cells and increases breast cancer cell detachment and invasive capacity (Queen et al. 2005). Neutrophils can mobilize angiogenic factors, such as VEGF, stored in the extracellular matrix through the release of MMP-9 (Nozawa et al. 2006). Expression of HPV 16 early region genes in basal keratinocytes of transgenic mice elicits a multi-stage pathway to squamous carcinoma. Infiltration by neutrophils and mast cells, and activation of MMP-9 in these cells coincided with the angiogenic switch in premalignant lesions (Coussens and Werb 1996). Lack of MMP-9 was associated with delayed activation of angiogenesis in the stroma of hyperplastic lesions (Coussens et al. 2000).

In the Rip-Tag2 model of pancreatic islet carcinogenesis, MMP-9-expressing neutrophils were predominantly found in the angiogenic islets of dysplasias and tumors, and transient depletion of neutrophils clearly reduced the frequency of the initial angiogenic switch in the dysplasias (Nozawa et al. 2006). The lack of both MMP-9-positive neutrophils and MMP-2-expressing-stromal cells in mice with a double deficiency for MMP-2 and MMP-9 resulted in a lack of tumor vascularization followed by a lack of tumor invasion (Masson et al. 2005). Expression of G-CSF or co-expression of G-CSF and GM-CSF together induced malignant progression of previously benign factor-negative HaCaT tumor cells. This progression was associated with enhanced and accelerated neutrophil recruitment into the tumor vicinity. The neutrophil recruitment preceded the induction of angiogenesis in the HaCaT heterotransplantation model for human squamous cell carcinoma and in nude mouse heterotransplants of head and neck carcinomas (Obermueller et al. 2004; Gutschalk et al. 2006).

In some tumors, like melanoma, neutrophils are not a major constituent of the leukocyte infiltrate, but they might have a key role in triggering and sustaining the inflammatory cascade, providing chemotactic molecules for the recruitment of macrophages and other inflammatory and stromal cells. Neutrophils produce and release high levels of MMP-9. By contrast, neutrophils secrete little, if any, MMP-2, which plays an important role in the turnover of various extracellular matrix components (Muhs et al. 2003). However, neutrophils release a not yet identified soluble factor as well as a specific sulphatase and a heparanase that activate latent MMP-2 secreted by other cells and allow releasing of embedded growth factors from the extracellular matrix (Schwartz et al. 1998; Bartlett et al. 1995). Remodeled matrix facilitates the escape of tumor cells leaving the tumor mass to metastasize at distance, because it offers less resistance. In addition, proteolytic enzymes released by neutrophils can diminish cell-cell interactions and permit the dissociation of tumor cells from the original tumor site (Shamamian et al. 2001). Gordon-Weeks et al. (2017) have demonstrated that neutrohils recruited into liver-metastatic microenvronment produce FGF-2, which induces tumor angiogenesis and metastasis. Moreover, a FGF-2 neutralizing antibody, when administered oneweek post tumor cell infiltration, induces a reduction of vascular density, cancer cell proliferation, and metastasis.

Human neutrophils synthesise and secrete small anti-microbial peptides known as alpha-defensins, which exert inhibition of endothelial cell proliferation, migration and adhesion, impaired capillary tube formation *in vitro*, and reduced angiogenesis *in vivo* (Chavakis et al. 2004). In addition, neutrophil-derived elastase can generate the anti-angiogenic factor angiostatin (Scapini et al. 2002) a well known inhibitor of IL-8-, macrophage inflammatory protein (MIP)-2- and growth-related oncogen alpha (GRO-alpha)-induced angiogenesis *in vivo* (Benelli et al. 2002). Remarkably, all-trans retinoic acid, a promising molecule with potential anti-angiogenic use in clinical treatment, has been shown to inhibit VEGF formation in cultured neutrophil-like HL-60 cells (Tee et al. 2006).

7.1.1   Neutrophils, Angiogenesis, and Inflammation

During the acute inflammatory response, neutrophils extravasate from the circulation into the tissue, where they exert their defence functions. Increasing evidence supports the concept that these immune cells also contribute to inflammation-mediated angiogenesis in different flogistic conditions.

Neutrophils indeed are a source of soluble mediators which, besides proinflammatory activity, exert important angiogenic functions. In this perspective, microarray technique has recently revealed about 30 angiogenesis-relevant genes in human polymorphonuclear granulocytes (Schruefer et al. 2006). Interestingly, neutrophil-derived VEGF can stimulate neutrophil migration (Ancelin et al. 2004). Thus neutrophil contribution to both normal and pathological angiogenesis may be sustained by an autocrine amplification mechanism that allows persistent VEGF release to occur at sites of neutrophil accumulation. Production and release of VEGF from neutrophils has been shown to depend from the G-CSF (Ohki et al. 2005). Evidence for the possible role of polymorphonuclear granulocytes in inflammation-mediated angiogenesis and tissue remodeling was initially provided by the finding that CXC receptor 2 (CXCR2)-deficient mice, which lacks neutrophil infiltration in thioglycollate-induced peritonitis (Cacalano et al. 1994), showed delayed angiogenesis and impaired cutaneous wound healing (Devalaraja et al. 2000). Moreover, human polymorphonuclear granulocytes have demonstrated the ability to directly induce the sprouting of capillary-like structures in *in vitro* angiogenesis assay. This angiogenic capacity appears to be mediated by secretion of both preformed VEGF from cell stores and *de novo* synthesized IL-8 (Schruefer et al. 2006).

Analysis of the synovium in patients with chronic pyogenic arthritis identified dramatic neovascularization and cell proliferation, accompanied by persistent bacterial colonization and heterogeneous inflammatory infiltrates rich in CD15[+] neutrophils, as histopathologic hallmarks (Pessler et al. 2008). By using a modified angiogenic model, allowing for a direct analysis of exogenously added cells and their products in collagen implants grafted on the chorioallantoic membrane of the chicken embryo, it has been demonstrated that intact human neutrophils and their granule contents are highly angiogenic (Ardi et al. 2007). Furthermore, purified neutrophil MMP-9, isolated from the released granules as a zymogen (proMMP-9), constitutes a distinctly potent proangiogenic moiety inducing angiogenesis at subnanogram levels. The angiogenic response induced by neutrophil proMMP-9 requires activation of the tissue inhibitor of metalloproteinases (TIMP)-free zymogen and the catalytic activity of the activated enzyme.

Neutrophils not only activate but also modulate the angiogenic process. Neutrophil elastase, a serine protease released from the azurophil granules of activated neutrophil, proteolytically cleaves angiogenic growth factors such as FGF-2 and VEGF (Ai et al. 2007). Neutrophil elastase degrades FGF-2 and VEGF in a time- and concentration-dependent manner, and these degradations are suppressed by sivelestat, a synthetic inhibitor of neutrophil elastase. The FGF-2- or VEGF-mediated proliferative activity of human umbilical vein endothelial cells is inhibited by neutrophil elastase, and the activity is recovered by sivelestat. Furthermore, neutrophil elastase reduces the FGF-2- or VEGF-induced tubulogenic response of the mice aortas, *ex vivo* angiogenesis assay, and these effects are also recovered by sivelestat.

7.2 Monocytes-Macrophages

Cells belonging to the monocyte-macrophage lineage are a major component of the leukocyte infiltration in tumors. It can reach up to 50% of the total mass (Balkwill and Mantovani 2001; Mantovani et al. 2002).

Macrophages are derived from CD34 positive bone marrow progenitors that continually proliferate and shed their progeny in the bloodstream as promonocytes. They then develop into monocyte and extravasate into tissues where they differentiate into a specific type of "resident" tissue macrophage (Fig. 7.2) (Ross and Auger 2002). If the bone marrow is destroyed by exposing an animal to X-rays, injury fail to elicit any mononuclear cell response, whereas if the thymus is removed a normal reponse is produced.

Elie Metchnikoff (Fig. 7.3) was the first person in 1893 to use the term "macrophage" to describe a large cell able to take up microorganisms (Tauber and Chernyak 1991). Aschoff identified these cells as macrophages in connective tissues, microglia in the central nervous system, endothelial cells lining vascular sinusoids, and reticular cells of lymphoid organs, and grouped these cells collectively into the reticuloendothelial system (RES).

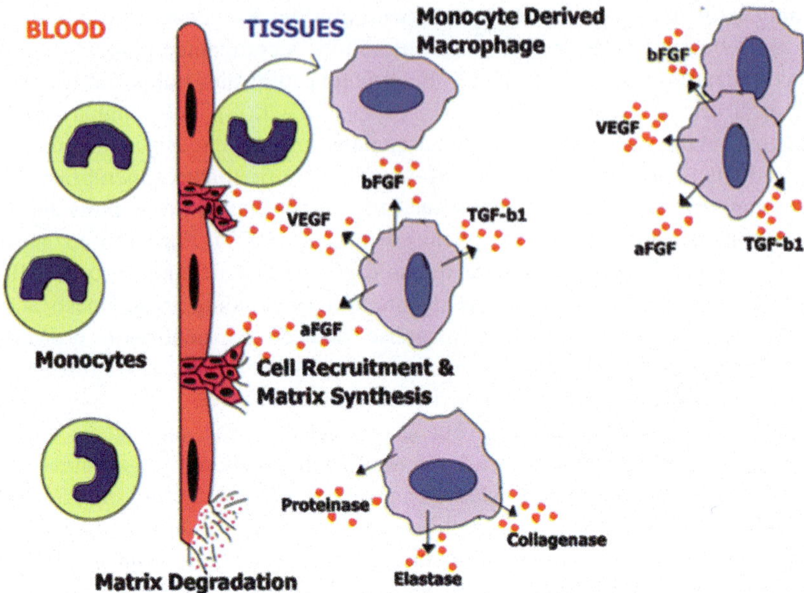

Fig. 7.2 After entering the peripheral blood, monocytes are recruited by chemokines into the tissue and undergo differentiation into macrophages. The specialization and activation of these cells are mainly influenced by local stimuli (Reproduced from Garg et al. 2009)

Fig. 7.3 A port trait of Elie Metchinkoff (from Wilkipidia)

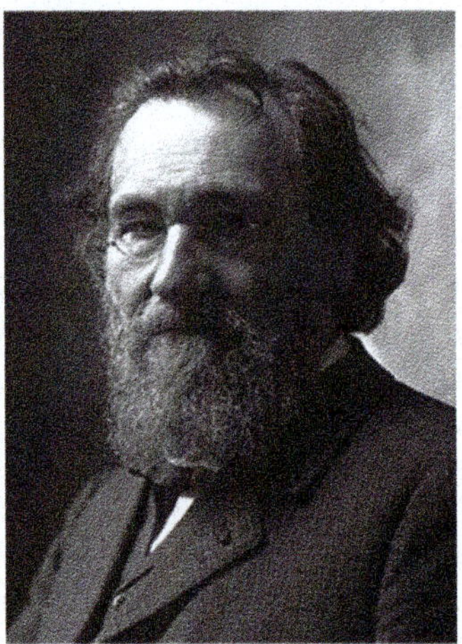

The phenotype of these fully differentiated, resident macrophages can vary markedly within tissues, from that of microglial cells in the brain, Kupffer cells in the liver, alveolar macrophages in the lung and Langherans cells in the skin. Resident macrophages share a set of common functions, including their ability to intervene against microbial infections, to regulate normal cell turnover and tissue remodeling, and to help repair sites of injury (Ross and Auger 2002). Besides killing tumor cells once activated by IFN-γ and IL-12, tumor-associated macrophages (TAMs) produce several pro-angiogenic cytokines as well as extracellular matrix-degrading enzymes (Naldini and Carraro 2005). Based on their phenotype and functions, both mouse and human monocytes can be divided in two main substets, "inflammatory" or "classical" monocytes, and "resident" or "non classical" monocytes (Geissmann et al. 2010). Whereas "inflammatory" monocytes can rapidly differentiate into macrophages or dendritic cells upon their extravasation, the role of "resident "monocytes is still poor understood. Monocytes release VEGF, CXCL3, COX-2, and MMP-9 to induce angiogenic response and are recruited to inflammatory sites through angiopoietin-2 (Ang-2) (Chambers et al. 2013). Recruited monocytes derived from the pool of circulating Ly6Chi monocytes undergo phenotypic and functional changes in a VEGF-rich environment, and acquire enhanced pro-angiogenic capabilities and the capacity to remodel existing blood vessels (Avraham-Davidi et al. 2013). The half-life of circulating monocytes is about 1 day; under the influence of adhesion molecules and chemotactic factors, they begin to emigrate at a site of injury within the first 24–48 h after onset of acute inflammation. An increased number of monocytes is associated with chronic diseases, including rheumatoid arthritis, liver chirrosis, tubercolosis, malaria and other chronic infections.

The granules of mature monocytes are much smaller than those of neutrophils and are barely visible by light microscopy. Phagocytosis of tumor cells by monocytes has been demonstrated and when placed on a surface to which they adhere, monocytes become indistinguishable from tissue macrophages by scanning electron microscopy.

The classical studies of Lewis and Lewis in 1926, Maximov in 1932, and Ebert and Florey in 1939, showed that monocytes transform into macrophages and multinucleated giant cells in vitro. Monocyte differentiated into polarized macrophage subset when exposed to different cytokine milieu (Sica et al. 2006). In the presence of GM-CSF, IFN-γ, LPS and other microbial products, monocyte differentiate into M1 macrophage. In the presence of macrophage colony stimulating factor (M-CSF), IL-4, IL-13, IL-10, immunosuppressive agents (corticosteroids, vitamin D3, prostaglandins) monocytes differentiate into M2 macrophages, involved in tumor angiogenesis. Both mouse and human tumors produce tumor-derived chemotactic factors capable of stimulating monocyte migration (Graves and Valente 1991).

Activated macrophages are generally categorized in two types, M1 (classically activated) and M2 (alternatively activated) (Fig. 7.4, Tables 7.4, and 7.5) (Balkwill and Mantovani 2001). The differentiation toward M1 and M2 activation states is regulated by defined substets of miRNA (O'Neill et al. 2011). MiR-126 suppresses the recruitment of inflammatory monocytes into the tumor stroma (Zhang et al. 2013), while overexpression of hypoxia-inducible miR-210 increases the recruitment of monocytes and their M2-macrophage polarization and the support of tumor angiogenesis (Taddei et al. 2014). M1 macrophages are considered to be proinflammatory and phagocytic, and are able to kill microorganisms as well as tumor cells and secrete high levels of pro-inflammatory cytokines, including IL-1β, IL-23, and proteases, and tumoricidal agents (TNF-α and IL-12), reactive nitrogen and oxygen intermediates (RNI, ROI), and low levels of anti-inflammatory IL-10 (Balkwill

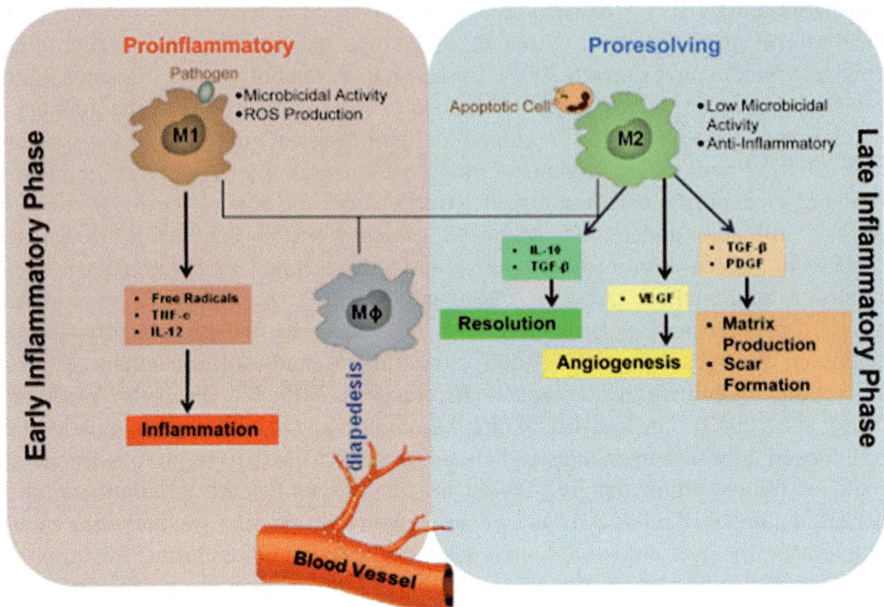

Fig. 7.4 In the early phase, the inflammatory milieu drives macrophage toward M1 polarization. M1 macrophages possess potent microbicidal properties and support IL-12-mediated type 1 helper T-cell responses. In the late inflammatory phase, the change in microenvironment drive the M1 macrophages toward M2 polarization. M2 supports type 2 helper T-cell-related effector functions. (Reproduced from Das et al. 2015)

Table 7.4 M1 and M2 macrophage fetarures and functions

M1 functions
Activate adaptive immune response through antigen presentation on upregulated MHC class II molecules
Produce reactive oxygen intermediates and nitric oxide for microbial killing
Produce solube VEGF receptor
M1 features vs M2
< IL-4; IL-10; > IL-6; > IL-12, IL-23; > TNFα.
M2 functions
Down-regulate adaptive immune response through down-regulation of MHC class II molecules
Secretion EGF/tumor invasion
Secretion of VEGF/angiogenesis
Secretion of MMPs
M2 features vs M1
< IL-12; >IL-10, IL-17; > TGF-β; activated STAT-3

Table 7.5 Factors influencing macrophage phenotype

Promote M1 phenotype
IFN-γ
LPS
GM-CSF
TNF-α
Lipothecoic acid
Promote M2 phenotype
CSF-1
Intracellular pathogens
M2a, IL-4, IL-13
M2b, immune complexes, Toll-like receptor; IL-1 receptor agonists.
M2c, IL-10; glucocorticoids
Promote M2/M1 swicth
GM-CSF
STAT3/STAT6 inhibitors
Anti-IL-4 anti-IL10 receptor antibodies.

et al. 2005). TNF-α kills tumor cells by at least two different mechanisms. First, binding of TNF to high-affinity cell surface receptors is directly toxic to tumor cells. Second, TNF can cause tumor necrosis by mobilizing various host responses in vivo.

Classically activated macrophages elicit antumor effects that are immunologically nonspecific in that they act upon tumor cells irrespective of species, but they are selective in that tumor cells are affected. In the tumor microenvironment, TAMs are mainly constituted by M2 elements (Mantovani et al. 2002), which produce a large amounts of arginase-1, IL-10 and VEGF, have poor attitude to destroy tumor cells but are better adapted to promoting angiogenesis, repairing and remodeling wounded or damaged tissues, and suppressing adaptive immunity (Sica et al. 2006). In regressing and non-progressing tumors, TAMs mainly resemble the M1 type and exhibit anti-tumor activity, while in malignant and advanced tumors, TAMs are biased toward the M2 phenotype that favors tumor malignancy (Qian and Pollard 2010). Unique cell surface markers that distinguish the two TAM phenotypes remain elusive and expression of M1/M-2 associated molecules is highly dependent on tumor type, tumor stage, intratumoral localization, hypoxia, and other microenvironmental signals (Mantovani et al. 2002). The phenotype of polarized M1-M2 macrophages has the potential to be reversed (Guiducci et al. 2005). Rolny et al. (2011) demonstrated that the host-produced histidine-rich glycoprotein (HRG) skewed TAM polarization away from the M2 to a tumor-inhibiting M1-like phenotype. In this context, HRG promoted antitumor immune responses and vessel normalization. Extensive TAM infiltration correlates with a poor prognosis for breast, prostate, cervix, and bladder cancer patients (Talmadge et al. 2007).

A relationship between the macrophage content ot tumors, the rate of tumor growth and the extent of their vascularization has been demonstrated in several tumors, including breast carcinoma where TAM presence focally in large numbers correlates with a high level of angiogenesis and with poor prognosis, decreased relapse-free and overall survival of the patients (Leek et al. 1996; Lee et al. 2002), B-cell non Hodgkin's lymphoma (Fig. 7.5) (Vacca et al. 1999), diffuse large B-cell lymphoma (Fig. 7.6) (Marinaccio et al. 2014), malignant uveal melanoma (Makitie et al. 2001), glioma (Nishie et al. 1999), squamous cell carcinoma of the esophagus (Koide et al. 2004), bladder carcinoma (Hanada et al. 2000) and prostate carcinoma (Lissbrant et al. 2000). In lung cancer, TAM may favour tumor progression by contributing to stroma formation and angiogenesis through their release of PDGF in conjunction with TGF-β-1 production by cancer cells (Mantovani et al. 2002).

In PyMT-induced mammary tumors, TAMs are recruited to pre-malignant lesions immediately before the onset of angiogenesis and then induce the angiogenic switch (Lewis and Pollard 2006).

Tumor-derived chemo attractants ensure macrophage recruitment, including CSF-1, the CC chemokines CCL-2, CCL-3, CCL-4, CCL-5 and CCL-8, and VEGF secreted by both tumor and stromal elements (Mantovani et al. 2002). TAMs derived from circulating monocytes and are recruited at the tumor site by a tumor-derived chemotactic factor from monocytes, originally described by Bottazzi et al. (1983), and later identified as the chemokine CCL2/MCP-1 (Matsushima et al. 1989; Yoshimura et al. 1989). When exposed to VEGF (Marumo et al. 1999) or to brief ischemia (Lakshminarayanan et al. 2001) endothelial cells synthesize MCP-1 and the extent of MCP-1 expression in human cancers correlated with both TAM infiltration and tumor malignancy in human melanoma, in Kaposi sarcoma cell lines and in human tumor cell lines of epithelial origin such as breast, colon and ovary (Ueno et al. 2000). Moreover, MCP-1 is angiogenic when implanted into the rabbit cornea, where it exerted a potency similar to VEGF (Goede et al. 1999). MCP-1 expression correlates significantly with levels of VEGF, TNF-α and IL-8 (Bingle et al. 2002; Varney et al. 2005; Liss et al. 2001). The expression of CCL5/RANTES is elevated in breast tumor cells synergistically by IFN-γ and TNF-α, regulating monocyte migration into tumor sites and stimulate them to secrete MMP-9 and MMP-19 (Locati et al. 2002; Azenshtein et al. 2002).

CSF and GM-CSF are commonly produced in a range of different tumor types and are chemotactic for macrophages *in vitro* (Dorsch et al. 1993). Transplanted mouse tumors transfected with the GM-CSF gene exhibit increased TAM infiltration (Heike et al. 1993) and genetic deletion of CSF-1 in the PyMT mouse model of breast cancer dramatically decreased TAM infiltration and attenuated tumor progression to metastasis (Lin et al. 2001). Elevated expression of GM-CSF has been found in human breast, endometrial and ovarian tumors (Kacinski 1995) and high GM-CSF expression is associated with high TAM accumulation in breast carcinomas (Tang et al. 1992). Also VEGF is chemotactic for monocytes via VEGFR-1 (Clauss et al. 1990; Leek et al. 2000).

The first evidence for a role of macrophages in angiogenesis was presented by Sunderkötter et al. 1991. TAMs express and release different pro- and anti-angiogenic molecules (Fig. 7.7), including EGF, FGF-2 (Baird et al. 1985; Joseph-Silverstein et al. 1988), TGF-α and TGF-β (Madtes et al. 1988; Rappolee et al. 1988; Assoian

Fig. 7.5 Comparison of microvessel and macrophage counts in multiple myeloma. Significance of the regression analysis was calculated by Pearson's r-test. LG, low-grade; IG, intermediate-grade; HG, high-grade (Reproduced from Vacca et al. 1999)

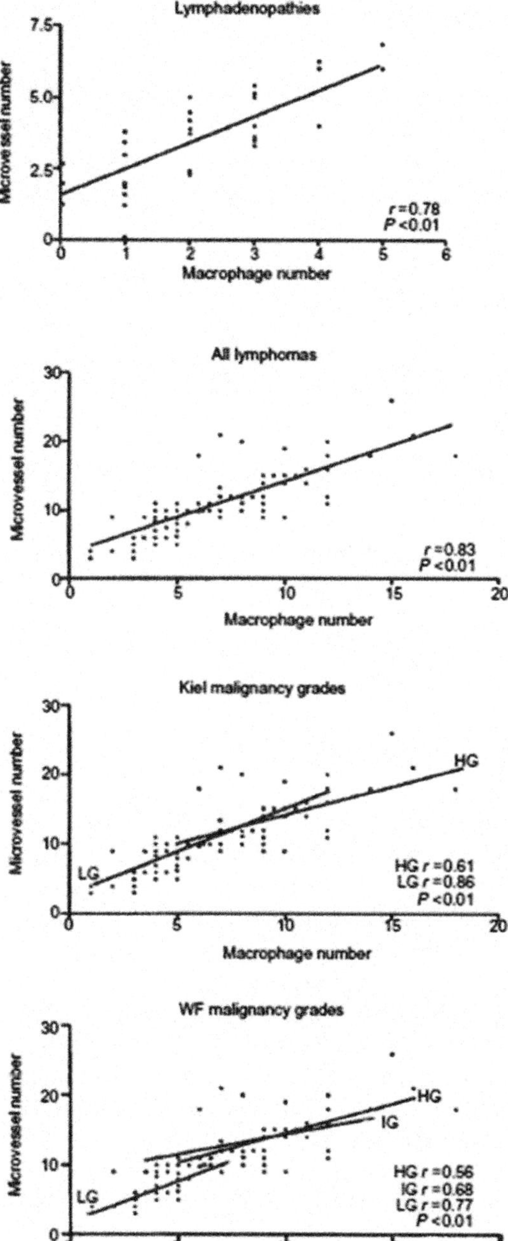

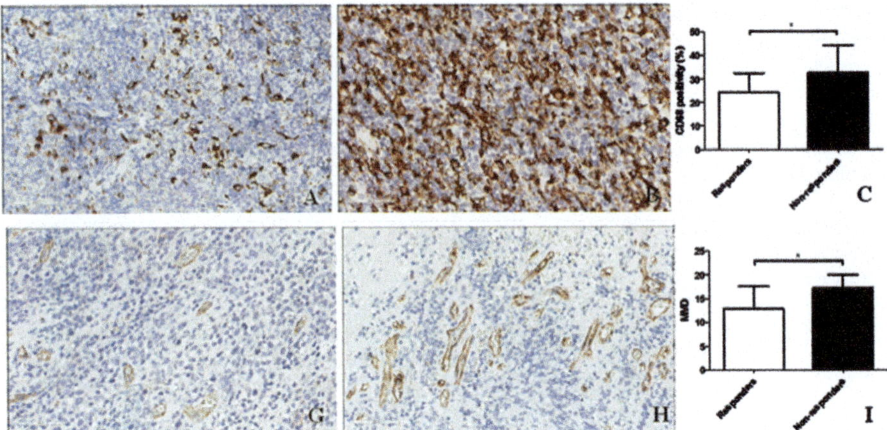

Fig. 7.6 CD68 and CD31 expression in responders and no-responder's groups of patients affected by Diffuse Large B-cell Lymphoma (DLBCL). (**a**) CD68 expression in a responder case. (**b**) CD68 expression in a non-responder case. (**c**) Comparison between responders and no-responder's groups with a significant difference between the groups in the expression of CD68. (**g**) CD31 for microvessel staining in a responder case. (**h**) CD31 for microvessel staining in a non-responder case. (**i**) Comparison between responders and no-responder's groups with a significant difference between the groups in microvascular density. *$p < 0.05$ (Modified from Marinaccio et al. 2014)

et al. 1987), VEGF (Berse et al. 1992), TNF-α (Leibovich et al. 1987), IL-1 (Roberts et al. 1986), IL-6, IL-8 (Koch et al. 1992), platelet activating factor (PAF) (Seo et al. 2004) PDGF (Martinet et al. 1986) G-CSF and GM-CSF (Sullivan et al. 1983), thymidine phosphorylase (TP) (Hotchkiss et al. 2003) and chemokines, such as CCL2 (Vicari and Caux 2002). TAMs produce, besides, angiogenic factors, angiostatic molecules such as thrombospondin-1 (Di Pietro and Polverini 1993), IL-12 (Inoue et al. 2005), IL-18 (Belardelli and Ferrantini 2003) and MMP-12 (Kerkela et al. 2000). TAMs are he major source of semaphorin 4D (sema 4D), a pro-angiogenic molecule that acts through its receptor, plexin B1 (Conrotto et al. 2005), which is critical for tumor angiogenesis (Sierra et al. 2008).

TAMs may also induce tissue remodeling by producing various proteinase activators and inhibitors that may destroy the integrity of the basement membrane and extracellular matrix, liberating matrix-bound factors, including MMP-2, MMP-9, MMP-7, MMP-12, and cycloxygenase-2 (COX-2) (Sunderkötter et al. 1991; Lewis et al. 1994; Klimp et al. 2001). TAM production of MMP-9 is crucial for angiogenesis in a human papillomavirus-16-induced model of cervical carcinogenesis. In this model inhibition of MMP-9 in macrophages blocked the release of VEGF and thereby inhibited angiogenesis and tumor growth (Giraudo et al. 2004). Inhibition of CSF-1 function in human tumors xenografted into immunocompromized mice reduced their growth and this was correlated with poor macrophage recruitment and reduced angiogenesis due to a depletion of VEGF.

Following hypoxia, circulating monocytes are recruited to the effected region and differentiate into macrophages. Monocyte recruitment to sites of hypoxia is

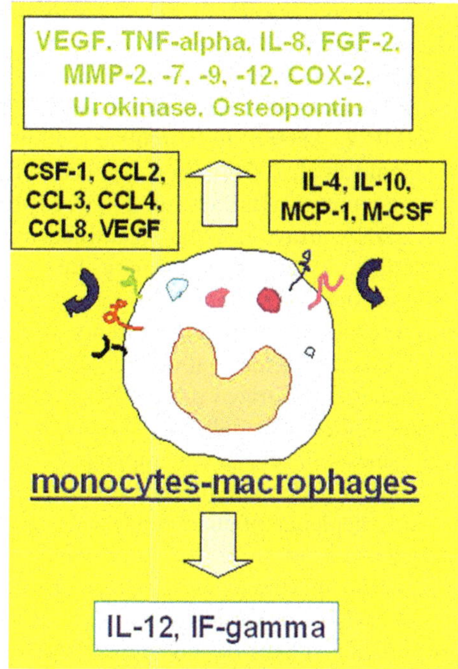

Fig. 7.7 Interplay between angiogenic and anti-angiogenic molecules secreted by monocytes-macrophages (Modified from Ribatti and Crivellato 2009)

driven by generation of pro-inflammatory signals (Shi and Pamer 2011). In human monocytes, hypoxia induced nuclear accumulation of HIF-1α in an NFkB dependent manner (Fangradt 2012). Differentiated macrophages require a priming stimulus (eg. LPS or IFNγ) in order to respond to hypoxia in a pro-inflammatory manner, while monocytes do not (Bosco et al. 2008).

TAMs accumulate in hypoxic regions of tumors and hypoxia triggers a pro-angiogenic program in these cells. TAMs adaptation to hypoxia, which is achieved by the increased expression of hypoxia inducible and pro-angiogenic genes, such as VEGF, FGF-2 and CXCL8, as well as glycolytic enzymes, whose transcriptions is controlled by the transcription factors HIF-1 and HIF-2 (Talks et al. 2000). Increased number of TAMs in hypoxic regions may promote tumor progression in part by stimulating levels of angiogenesis, such as occurs in breast carcinoma (Leek et al. 1999). Up-regulation of the pro-angiogenic program in tumor-associated macrophages, followed by increased release of VEGF, FGF-2, TNF-α, urokinase and MMPs, is stimulated by hypoxia and acidosis (Bingle et al. 2002). White et al. (2004) used adenoviral infection to overexpress HIF-2 in human macrophages and found it to be the primary inducer of genes encoding angiogenic cytokines in these genes. Macrophages also up-regulates VEGF and other proangiogenic factors in response to hypoxia. Mice deficient in HIF-2α in myeloid cells, displayed reduced TAM infiltration in both murine hepatocellular and colitis-associated colon carcinoma models (Imtiyaz et al. 2010). Moreover, in mouse mammary tumors, exhibiting enriched M2-like TAMs in hypoxic tumor areas, demonstrated an increased pro-angiogenic phenotype *in vivo*, with numbers elevating as the tumor progressed (Movahedi et al. 2010).

TAMs express VEGF almost exclusively in avascular and perinecrotic areas of human breast carcinoma (Lewis et al. 2000). TAMs also synthesize elevated levels of MMP-7, known to stimulate endothelial cell proliferation and migration (Nishizuka et al. 2001), when exposed to hypoxia *in vitro* and in an avascular areas of human tumors (Burke et al. 2003). MMP-7 is.

A cDNA array study has identified up-regulation of messanger encoding >30 proangiogenic genes in primary macrophages exposed to hypoxia, including CXCL8, Ang, COX-2 and other factors (White et al. 2004). When macrophages are cocultured in vitro with human tumor spheroids, they infiltrate deep into the central, hypoxic areas of these structures (Bingle et al. 2005). The release of VEGF by macrophages-infiltrated spheroids was significantly higher than that seen for noninfiltrated spheroids, and this increase translated into a significant stimulation of angiogenesis *in vivo* when implanted into microcirculation window chambers on the flanjs of nude mice for 3 days (Bingle et al. 2005).

Mice depleted of macrophages by whole-body X-irradiation or azathioprine administered before or after implantation of a syngeneic fibrosarcoma showed a delay in the appearance of tumors, and a marked reduction in tumor vascularization (Evans 1977a, b). Vascularization of several human tumor cell lines grown on the chick embryo CAM or subcutaneously in nude mice occurred coincidentally with mononuclear cell infiltration at the tumor site (Mostafa et al. 1980a, b; Stenzinger et al. 1982).

Polverini and Leibovich (1984) isolated macrophages from a transplantable rat fibrosarcoma and examined them and their serum free conditioned media for angiogenic activity in rat corneas. Results showed that TAMs and their conditioned media were potently angiogenic *in vivo* and stimulated proliferation of bovine aortic endothelial cells in culture. Moreover, when TAMs were combined with tumor cells at a concentration equivalent to the number of macrophages originally present in the tumor there was a marked enhancement of tumor neovascularization and growth. Moreover, hamsters bearing chemical carcinogen-induced squamous cell carcinomas showed a marked reduction in the thymidine incorporation by endothelial cells and neovascularization of tumors when treated with low doses of steroids and anti-macrophage serum (Polverini and Leibovich 1987).

In the mouse model of breast cancer caused by the mammary epithelial cell restricted expression of the Polyoma middle T oncoprotein (PyMT mice) infiltration of TAMs in primary tumors is positively associated with tumor progression to malignancy (Lin et al. 2001). Depletion of macrophages in this model severely delayed tumor progression and reduced metastasis, whereas an increase in macrophage infiltration remarkably accelerated these processes. By using the PyMT-induced mouse mammary tumors, Lin et al. (2006) characterized the development of the vasculature in mammary tumors during their progression to malignancy. They demonstrated that both angiogenic switch and the progression to malignancy are regulated by infiltrated macrophages in the primary mammary tumors. Moreover, inhibition of the macrophage infiltration into the tumor delayed the angiogenic switch and malignant transition, whereas genetic reduction of the macrophage population specifically in these tumors rescued the vessel phenotype. Finally, premature induction of macrophage infiltration into premalignant lesions promoted an early onset of the angiogenic switch independent of tumor progression (Lin et al. 2006).

Lewis lung carcinoma cells expressing IL-1-β develop neo-vasculature with macrophage infiltration and enhance tumor growth in wild-type but not in MCP-1-deficient mice, suggesting that macrophage involvement might be a prerequisite for neovascularization and tumor progression (Nakao et al. 2005).

Activated macrophages synthesize and release inducible nitric oxide synthase, which increases blood flow and promotes angiogenesis (Jenkins et al. 1995). The angiogenic factors secreted by macrophages stimulate migration of other accessory cells that potentiate angiogenesis, in particular mast cells (Gruber et al. 1995). Osteopontin deeply affects the pro-angiogenic potential of human monocytes (Denhardt et al. 2001), and may affect angiogenesis by acting directly on endothelial cells and/or indirectly via mononuclear phagocyte engagement, enhancing the expression of TNF-α and IL-1-β in mononuclear cells (Leali et al. 2003; Naldini et al. 2006).

Macrophages produce IL-12, which cause tumor regression and reduce metastasis in animal models, through the promotion of anti-tumor immunity and also to the significant inhibition of angiogenesis (Colombo and Trinchieri 2002). The anti-angiogenic activity is mediated by IFN-γ production, which in turn induces the chemokine IFN-γ-inducible protein-10 (Romagnani et al. 2001). Moreover, IL-12 inhibits VEGF production by breast cancer cells and regulates stromal cell interactions, leading to decreased MMP-9 and increased tissue inhibitor of TIMP-1 production (Dias et al. 1998).

Using PyMT mice, Lin et al. (2007) demonstrated that both the angiogenic switch and the progression to malignancy are regulated by infiltrated macrophages. Moreover, inhibition of macrophage homing into the tumor microenvironment delayed the angiogenic switch, whereas genetic restoration of macrophages rescued the vascular phenotype.

The developing vasculature in tumors lacking myeloid-cell-derived VEGF-A was less tortuous, with increased pericyte coverage (indicating increased maturation), decreased vessel length, with evidence of vascular normalization and increased susceptibility to chemotherapeutic agents (Stockmann et al. 2008).

7.2.1 Monocytes/Macrophages, Angiogenesis, and Inflammation

Sarcoidosis is a systemic granulomatous inflammatory disease characterized by recruitment and activation of peripheral blood mononuclear cells to the sites of disease. It has been shown that sera from sarcoidosis patients enhance angiogenic capability of normal peripheral human mononuclear cells significantly stronger than sera from healthy donors (Zielonka et al. 2007). Angiogenic activity of sera in sarcoidosis depends on the stage of disease and appears most pronounced in stage

II. In addition, sera from patients with extrapulmonary changes exert stronger effect on angiogenesis than sera from patients with thoracic changes only. IL-6 and IL-8 serum level correlates with each other, but no correlation is observable between IL-6 and IL-8 serum level and angiogenic activity of the examined sera. Removal of monocytes from peripheral human mononuclear cells eliminates the effect of sera from sarcoidosis patients on angiogenesis compared with the effect of these sera on intact peripheral human mononuclear cells. Sera from sarcoidosis patients prime monocytes for production of proangiogenic factors.

There is accumulating evidence that delivery of bone marrow cells to sites of ischemia by direct local injection or mobilization into the blood can stimulate angiogenesis. This has stimulated tremendous interest in the translational potential of angiogenic cell population(s) in the bone marrow to mediate therapeutic angiogenesis. It has been shown that the inflammatory subset of monocytes is selectively mobilized into blood after surgical induction of hindlimb ischemia in mice and is selectively recruited to ischemic muscle (Capoccia et al. 2008). Adoptive-transfer studies show that delivery of a small number of inflammatory monocytes early (within 48 h) of induction of ischemia results in a marked increase in the local production of MCP-1, which in turn, is associated with a secondary, more robust wave of monocyte recruitment. Studies of mice genetically deficient in MCP-1 or CCR2 indicate that although not required for the early recruitment of monocytes, the secondary wave of monocyte recruitment and subsequent stimulation of angiogenesis are dependent on CCR2 signaling. Collectively, these data suggest a role for MCP-1 in the inflammatory, angiogenic response to ischemia.

Healing of myocardial infarction requires monocytes/macrophages. These mononuclear phagocytes likely degrade released macromolecules and aid in scavenging of dead cardiomyocytes, while mediating aspects of granulation tissue formation and remodeling. It has also been recognized that distinct monocyte subsets contribute in specific ways to myocardial ischemic injury in mouse myocardial infarction. Two distinct phases of monocyte participation after myocardial infarction have been identified (Nahrendorf et al. 2007). Infarcted hearts modulate their chemokine expression profile over time, and they sequentially and actively recruit Ly-6C(hi) and -6C(lo) monocytes via CCR2 and CX(3)CR1, respectively. Ly-6C(hi) monocytes dominate early (phase I) and exhibit phagocytic, proteolytic, and inflammatory functions. Ly-6C(lo) monocytes dominate later (phase II), have attenuated inflammatory properties, and express vascular-endothelial growth factor. Consequently, Ly-6C(hi) monocytes digest damaged tissue, whereas Ly-6C(lo) monocytes promote healing via myofibroblast accumulation, angiogenesis, and deposition of collagen. Myocardial infarction in atherosclerotic mice with chronic Ly-6C(hi) monocytosis results in impaired healing, underscoring the need for a balanced and coordinated response.

A role for inflammation in modulating the extent of angiogenesis has been shown for systemic angiogenesis of the lung after left pulmonary artery ligation in a mouse model of chronic pulmonary thromboembolism. Depletion of neutrophils do not alter the angiogenic outcome, but blood flow to the left lung is significantly reduced after dexamethasone (general anti-inflammatory) treatment compared with untreated control left pulmonary artery ligation mice and significantly increased in T/B lymphocyte-deficient mice (Wagner et al. 2008). Adoptive transfer of splenocytes (T/B lymphocytes) significantly reverses the degree of angiogenesis observed in the Rag-1(−/−) (T/B lymphocyte deficient) mice back to the level of control left pulmonary artery ligation. These findings indicate that inflammatory cells modulate the degree of angiogenesis in this lung model where lymphocytes appear to limit the degree of neovascularization, whereas monocytes/macrophages likely promote angiogenesis.

Shear stress regulates the angiogenic potential of endothelial cells *in vitro* by an Ang-2-dependent mechanism (Tressel et al. 2008). The pathophysiological significance of this mechanism *in vivo* has been clarified in that Ang-2 plays an important role in blood flow recovery after arterial occlusion by regulating angiogenesis and arteriogenesis. In fact, C57Bl/6 J mice subjected to femoral artery ligation and injected with a specific Ang-2 inhibitor, L1–10, show a blunted blood flow recovery. L1–10, indeed, decreases smooth muscle cell coverage of neovessels without affecting capillary density, suggesting a specific role for Ang-2 in arteriogenesis. Ang-2 likely operates through monocyte activation. L1–10 decreases expression of intercellular and vascular cell adhesion molecules as well as infiltrating monocytes/macrophages in the ischemic tissue. Although L1–10 has no effect on the number of CD11b + cells (monocytes/macrophages) mobilized in the bone marrow, it maintains elevated numbers of circulating CD11b + cells in the peripheral blood. Thus, these results suggest that Ang-2 induces in ischemic tissue plays a critical role in blood flow recovery by stimulating inflammation and arteriogenesis.

Monocytes are one of the initial cell types to be recruited to a wound, in the context of fibrin clot invasion. Evidence has indicated additional involvement of Ang-2 in vascular homeostatic responses such as coagulation and inflammation, which are central to wound healing. Ang-2 significantly increased monocyte invasion of fibrin in the presence of serum. In the absence of serum, it required a combination of Ang-2 and platelet-derived growth factor BB (PDGF-BB) to increase invasion by threefold. Furthermore, it was shown that the heightened invasion was dependent on serine proteases and MMPs and that the combination of Ang-2 and PDGF-BB increased urokinase plasminogen-activator receptor expression, as well as MMP-9 and membrane type 1 MMP expression. These data give further credence to the concept of Ang-2 as a key regulator of several essential phases of wound healing (Bezuidenhout et al. 2007).

Monocyte-macrophage activation by IFN-γ is a key initiating event in inflammation. Usually, the macrophage response is self-limiting and inflammation resolves. A mechanism has been described by which IFN-γ contributes to inflammation resolution by suppressing expression of VEGF-A. Although IFN-γ induced persistent VEGF-A mRNA expression, translation is suppressed by delayed binding of the IFN-γ-activated inhibitor of translation complex to a specific element delineated in the 3'UTR. Translational silencing results in decreased VEGF-A synthesis and angiogenic activity. In addition, it contributes to inflammation resolution.

In atherosclerotic plaque, the transcription factor HIF-1α is associated with an atheromatous inflammatory plaque phenotype and with VEGF expression (Vink et al. 2007). Remarkably, HIF-1α expression is upregulated in activated macrophages under normoxic conditions. Hypoxia in advanced human atherosclerosis and its correlation with the presence of macrophages and the expression of HIF and VEGF (Sluimer et al. 2008). The HIF pathway was associated with lesion progression and angiogenesis, suggesting its involvement in the response to hypoxia and the regulation of human intraplaque angiogenesis.

Almost any local disturbance of tissue normality, be it infection, normal cell turnover or wounding, immune response or malignancy, caused rapid recruitment of macrophages. Recruited macrophages exhibit many phenotypic differences from resident tissue macrophages. The generic term, "macrophages activation" is commonly used to describe this process, but the nature of an "activated macrophage" population depends upon both the nature of the recruiting stimulus and the location.

It is now well established that the functional domain of the macrophage extends far beyond its originally recognized role as a scavenger cell. Its rich array of secretory products, anatomic diversity and functional heterogeneity is unmatched by any other cell type. As a result of this remarkable versatility, the macrophage is able to influence every facet of the immune response and inflammation as well as playing a central role in the etiology and/or pathogenesis of a number of disease processes.

7.2.2   Transdifferentation of Monocytes/Macrophages in Endothelial Cells and Tie-2 Monocytes

Monocytes/macrophages display a high degree of plasticity, as demonstrated by their ability to transdifferentiate into endothelial cells *in vitro* and *in vivo* (Fernandez Pujol et al. 2000; Rehman et al. 2003; Urbich et al. 2003; Schmeisser et al. 2001; Elsheikh et al. 2005; Fujiyama et al. 2003; Iba et al. 2002; Nowak et al. 2004; Zhao et al. 2003). CD14$^+$ mononuclear cells have been used as the starting population for cultivation of EPCs (Fernandez Pujol et al. 2000). Cultivated EPC grown from different starting populations, including peripheral blood mononuclear cells, express endothelial markers, including von Willebrand factor, VEGFR-2, VE-cadherin, CD156 and CD31 (Kalka et al. 2000). Monocytes coexpress endothelial lineage markers such as VEGFR-2 and AC133 and differentiate into adherent endothelial cells and form cord-like structures in Matrigel (Schmeisser et al. 2001, 2003). Bone marrow mononuclear cells contain not only EPC but also angiogenic factors and cytokines and implantation of bone marrow mononuclear cells into ischemic tissues augments collateral vessel formation (Kamihata et al. 2001; Shintani et al. 2001).

Peripheral blood monocytes CD14$^+$ and VEGFR-2$^+$ differentiate *in vitro* into cells with endothelial characteristics. Moreover, these cells transduced by a lentiviral vector driving expression of green fluorescent protein (GFP) and transplanted into ballon-injured femoral arteries of nude mice significantly centributed to efficient reendothelization (Elsheikh et al. 2005). Peripheral-blood endothelial-like cells derived from monocytes/macrophages and secrete angiogenic factors (Rehman et al. 2003).

Multiple myeloma bone marrow TAMs exposed to VEGF and FGF-2 develop a number of phenotypic properties similar to those of paired bone marrow endothelial cells, and form capillary-like structures overlapping morphologically those produced by endothelial cells (Scavelli et al. 2008). At ultrastructural level, multiple myeloma TAMs exhibit numerous cytoplasmic extroversions arranged in tube-like structures and these data suggest that TAMs contribute to build neovessels in multiple myeloma through vasculogenic mimicry (Scavelli et al. 2008).

7.2.3   Therapeutic Strategies

Macrophage itself become an appealing target for future anti-angiogenic therapeutic strategies through two approaches: compounds that suppress secretion of angiogenic substances by macrophages, and compounds that inhibit macrophage infiltration into the tumor mass.

Clodronate-liposomes depleted macrophages in the synovial fluid of rheumatoid arthritis patients and inhibited tumor angiogenesis in mouse tumor transplantation models (Barrera et al. 2000; Zeisberger et al. 2006). In the mouse cornea model, killing of COX-2 positive infiltrating macrophages with clodronate liposomes reduces IL-1-β-induced angiogenesis and partially inhibits VEGF-induced angiogenesis (Nakao et al. 2005).

VEGF inhibitors decrease macrophage recruitment, and this effect may contribute to their anti-angiogenic activity (Giraudo et al. 2004). Specific inhibition of VEGFR-2 decreased tumor macrophage infiltration into orthotopic pancreatic tumors (Dineen et al. 2008).

CSF-1 receptor (CSF-1R) kinase inhibitors exhibit anti-angiogenic and anti-metastatic activity in tumors (Manthey et al. 2009). Anti-CSF-1 antibodies and anti-sense oligonucleotides suppress macrophage infiltration and xenograft tumor growth in mice (Ahazinejad et al. 2002, 2004). Blockade of macrophage recruitment with CSF-1R-signalling antagonists in combination with paclitaxel decreased vessel density, reduced tumor growth and pulmonary metastasis, and improved survival of mammary tumor-bearing mice (De Nardo et al. 2011).

The broad elimination of TAMs by clodronate liposomes or CSF-1R antibodies, decreased angiogenesis in different tumor models (Zeisberger et al. 2006; Priceman et al. 2010; Lohela et al. 2014).

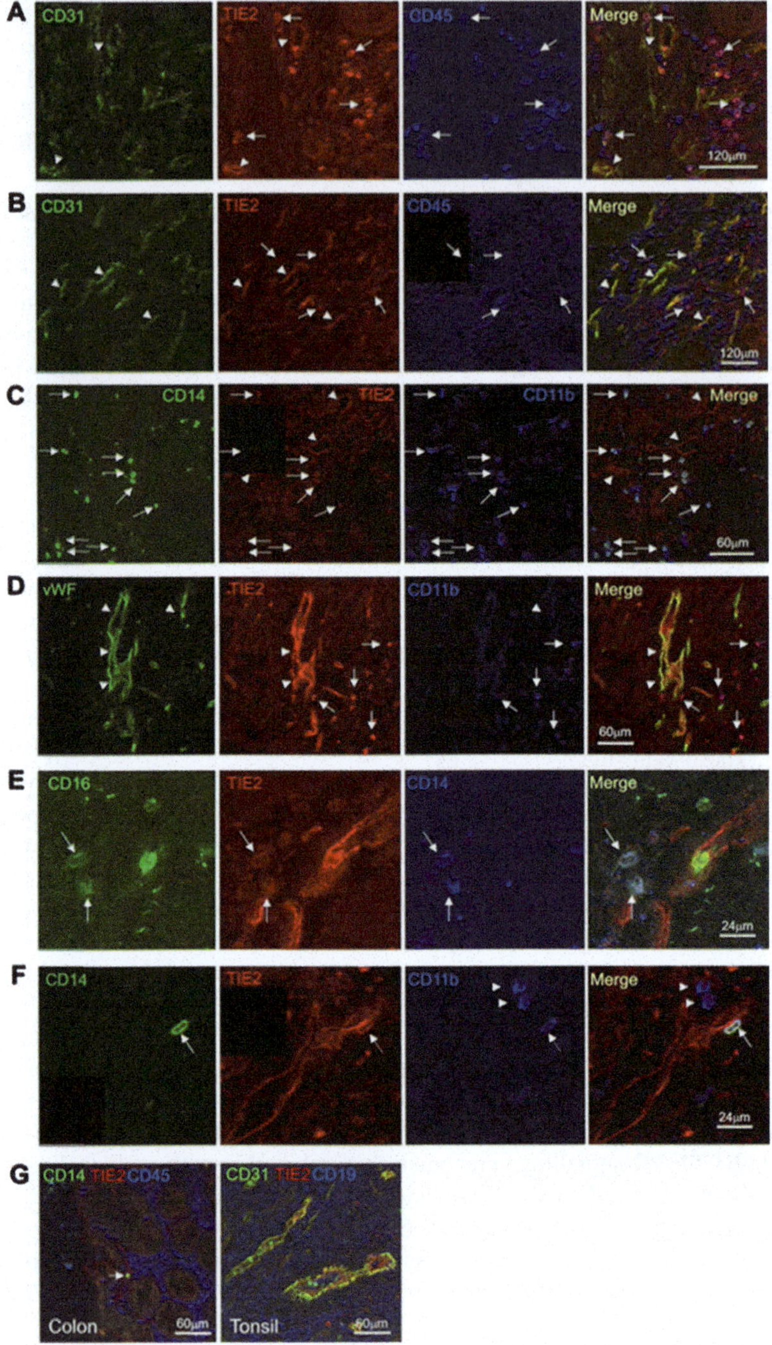

Fig. 7.8 **Confocal immunofluorescence analysis of human cancer sections confirms the presence of Tie-2[+]CD45[+]CD14[+]tumor-infiltrating monocytes**. (a) Colon adenocarcinoma analyzed for CD31 (green), Tie-2 (red), and CD45 (blue). Several Tie-2[+]CD45[+]CD31[−]hematopoietic cells (merge of red and blue giving purple; arrows) are found within the tumor stroma. Note that Tie-2 is expressed by vascular endothelial cells (merge of green and red giving yellow; arrowheads),

7.3   Tie-2 Expressing Monocytes (TEMs)

De Palma and collaborators identified a subpopulation of monocytes expressing the Tie-2 receptor (Tie-2 expressing monocytes, TEMs). Tie2 is a tyrosine kinase receptor broadly expressed in endothelial cells, involved in the regulation of angiogenesis and vascular morphogenesis both in development and adulthood (Augustin et al. 2009).

TEMs have been observed in several mouse tumor models, including subcutaneous tumor grafts, spontaneous insulinomas developing in RIP-TAG2 transgenic mice, and human gliomas growing in the mouse brain (De Palma et al. 2005). In these tumors, TEMs constituted a small population of the total tumor infiltrating CD11b$^+$ myeloid cells that could be distinguished from the majority of TAMs by their surface marker profile (Tie-2$^+$, Sca-1$^+$, CD11b$^+$) and their pro-angiogenic activity (De Palma et al. 2005). TEMs were found in human tumors including those of kidney, colon, pancreas and lung, as well as in soft tissue sarcomas, where angiogenesis is correlated to tumor progression (Fig. 7.8) (Venneri et al. 2007). In human cancer specimens, TEMs were found both in perivascular and hypoxic areas of tumors and were missing in non-neoplastic tissues adjacent to tumors (Venneri et al. 2007). Exposure to both hypoxia and Ang-2 markedly suppressed the release of an antiangiogenic cytokine, namely IL-12 (De Palma et al. 2003), and of TNF-α, which exterts a pro-apoptotic effect on both tumor cells and endothelial cells (Balkwill 1992). These data suggest that when monocytes are recruited into tumors and are exposed to both Ang-2 and hypoxia, they inhibit their ability to exert an antiangiogenic activity. Moreover, TNF-α down-regulation could enhance tumor and endothelial cell survival and thus promote metastasis and angiogenesis, respectively.

In a Tie-2 transgenic mouse model, TEMs were found in close proximity to endothelial cells, where they expressed high levels of FGF-2 (De Palma et al. 2005), but

Fig. 7.8 (continued) which are Tie-2$^+$CD45$^-$CD31$^+$. (**b**) Gastric adenocarcinoma analyzed for CD31 (green), Tie-2 (red), and CD45 (blue). Some Tie-2$^+$CD45$^+$CD31$^-$hematopoietic cells are found in the tumor stroma (arrows) together with Tie-2$^+$CD45$^-$CD31$^+$tumor blood vessels (arrowhead). (**c**) Colon adenocarcinoma analyzed for CD14 (green), Tie-2 (red), and CD11b (blue). Several Tie-2$^+$CD14$^+$CD11b$^+$monocytes (arrows) are found within the tumor stroma. Note Tie-2 expression by Tie-2$^+$CD14$^-$CD11b$^-$vascular endothelial cells (arrowheads). (**d**) Gastric adenocarcinoma analyzed for von Willebrand factor (green), Tie-2 (red), and CD11b (blue). Arrowheads indicate Tie-2$^+$CD11b$^+$VWF$^-$monocytes. (**e**) Pancreatic adenocarcinoma analyzed for CD16 (green), Tie-2 (red), and CD14 (blue). High-magnification photos show the presence of Tie-2$^+$CD16$^+$CD14$^+$monocytes (arrows) in the tumor stroma. (**f**) Colon adenocarcinoma analyzed for CD14 (green), Tie-2 (red), and CD11b (blue). A triple-positive CD14$^+$Tie-2$^+$CD11b$^+$TEM with peri-endothelial localization is indicated by the arrow. Note the presence of CD14$^-$Tie-2$^-$CD11b$^+$ inflammatory cells (arrowheads). (**g**) Tie-2 expression in no neoplastic tissues is restricted to vascular endothelial cells. Non neoplastic colon mucosa adjacent to tumor tissue analyzed by confocal immunofluorescence staining of CD31 or CD14 (green), Tie-2 (red), and CD45 (blue). Note that the lamina propria macrophages are CD14$^-$Tie-2$^-$. A single CD14$^+$Tie-2$^-$monocyte (arrow) is found within a Tie-2$^+$blood vessel. Tonsil sections show that Tie-2 expression (red) is restricted to CD31$^+$vascular endothelial cells (green). CD19$^+$B cells are stained in blue (Reproduced from Venneri et al. 2007)

not incorporated into nascent tumor vessels. Moreover, they did not differentiate into endothelial cells, suggesting that their pro-angiogenic activity could consist of a paracrine stimulation of angiogenesis. The selective elimination of TEMs by means of a suicide gene drammatically impaired angiogenesis in mouse tumors and induced substantial tumor regression (De Palma et al. 2003, 2005). In these tumor models, TEMs elimination did not affect the overall number of TAMs and granulocytes, indicating that TEMs represent a distinct monocyte subset with specific pro-angiogenic activity, which is primarily responsible for promoting angiogenesis. Moreover, although recruited to tumors in lower numbers than TAMs, TEMs are a more potent source of pro-angiogenic signals, suggesting that they significantly contribute to tumor angiogenesis.

These data indicate that while the concept of immature vascular cells delivered to the site of tumor blood vessels was originally developed on EPCs, it is become evident that other classes of vascular cells differentiate form progenitors *in situ*. The percentage of incorporated EPCs into tumor vessels is very low. TEMs, while stimulating angiogenesis, do not actively incorporate into blood vessels and this subpopulation of Tie-2$^+$ cells, rather than bone marrow-derived EPCs, which are incorporated in new-forming blood vessels, promote tumor neovascularization through the release of of pro-angiogenic factors (De Palma et al. 2003). TEMs may also play a role in angiogenesis in wound healing and in non-neoplastic diseases. In mice underwent partial hepatectomy 7–10 days earlier, TEMs were found in granulation tissue surrounding the regenerating hepatic lobules, also in proximity of newly-formed vessels, suggesting that they might also contribute to promoting angiogenesis during liver regeneration (De Palma et al. 2003).

TEMs were not observed in normal tissues suggesting that they may represent a specific subset of resident monocytes (Venneri et al. 2007). The identification of specific molecules expressed by TEMs in tumors could facilitate the design of novel anticancer therapies that selectively target these cells. De Palma et al. (2008), by transplanting hematopoietic progenitors transduced with a Tie-2 promoter/enhancer-driven IFN-α-1 gene, turned TEMs into IFN-α cell vehicles that targeted the IFN response to orthotopic human gliomas and spontaneous mouse mammary carcinomas and obtained significant antitumor responses and near complete abrogation of metastasis.

The extent each of the categories of bone marrow derived cells (BMDCs) contributes to tumor angiogenesis is currently not well defined. A very small number of EPCs can control the angiogenic switch in a mouse lung metastasis model (Gao et al. 2008). Their findings raise the question whether a small number of these angiogenic progenitor cells might have been present in the other transgenic mouse transplant model (Seandel et al. 2008). Phenotypic definition of BMDCs and EPCs that are present in tumor tissues are difficult to perform especially when the latter cell components are in small numbers. Perhaps all of the three categories of BMDCs contribute to tumor angiogenesis at different time of tumor development and location within the tumor microenvironment. Further elucidation of how the tumor angiogenic process is co-ordinated resides in a systematic testing and analysis of the biological mediators secreted by the BMDCs in the various tumor models.

TEMs are selectively recruited to spontaneous and orthotopic tumors; promote angiogenesis in a paracrine manner, and account for the majority of pro-angiogenic activity induced by myeloid cells in these tumors. Moreover, TEM knockout completely prevented human glioma neovascularization in the mouse brain and induced tumor regression without affecting the recruitment of TAMs or neutrophils into these tumors (De Palma et al. 2005), and their gene expression profile was highly related to TAMs (Pucci et al. 2009). Ang-2 (a Tie-2 ligand) blockade did not inhibit recruitment of TEMs to the tumor microenvironment, but abrogated their up-regulation of Tie-2 expression, association with blood vessels, and their ability to restore angiogenesis in tumors (Mazzieri et al. 2011). TEMs express MMP-9, VEGF, COX-2, WNT5A, and are localized in close proximity of blood vessels and to hypoxic areas of tumors (De Palma et al. 2005). Moreover, tumor TEMs mostly reside in viable and angiogenic tumor areas, whereas they are excluded from necrotic, inner tumor areas (De Palma and Naldini 2009). TEM-like pro-angiogenic monocytes/macrophages have been generated from human embryonic stem cells (Klimchenko et al. 2011).

7.4 Lymphocytes

Lymphocytes and plasma cells first were described in 1774 and 1875, repectively. By mid twentieth century, was established that immune system had at least two components, one governing cellular immunity and one governing humoral immunity. At the same time, it was discovered that the thymus and the bursa of Fabricius in birds were the source of T (thymic-derived) and B (bursa-derived) lymphocytes, respectively, and that bone marrow was the bursa equivalent in humans.

The lymphocytes consist of heterogeneous populations of cells that differ greatly from each other in terms of orign, life span, distribution within the lymphoid organs, surface structure, and function. The CD43 surface marker is expressed on human hematopoietic stem cells and on a variety of different types of hematopietic progenitors, including those restricted to the lymphoid development. Activation of B and T lymphocytes results in the transformation of the small, resting lymphocytes, into proliferating large cells with abundant highly basophilic cytoplasm, irregularly condensed chromatin, and round to slightly irregular nuclear outlines. Plasma cells derive from small B lymphocytes and their characteristic feature is abundant cytopalsmatic and secretory immunoglobulins.

B lymphocytes comprise 10–20% of the circulating peripheral lymphocyte population. B cells recognize antigen via monomeric surface IgM, the so-called B cell receptor, and the presence of rearranged immunoglobulin genes in a lymphoid cell is used as a molecular marker of B-lineage cells. High number of B cells have been found at the inflammatory sites in tumor tissues of various human cancer (Nelson 2010).

B cells express different pro-angiogenic mediators, including VEGF, FGF-2, and MMP-9 and B promote tumor progression via STAT3 regulated angiogenesis (Yang et al. 2013). Moreover, B-cell produced antibodies activate FCR gamma on both tumor–resident and recruited myeloid cells, which, in turn, recruite myofibroblasts in the tumor site which promote tumor angiogenesis (Andreu et al. 2010). In a mouse model of skin cancer, deposition of B cell-derived immunoglobulins in the skin recruits and activates pro-tumoral and pro-angiogenic TAMs (Andreu et al. 2010).

T cells constitute 60–70% of the lymphocytes in circulating blood and each T cell is genetically programmed to recognize a unique peptide fragment by means of a specific T-cell receptor (TCR).

T lymphocytes provide effective anti-tumor immunity in vivo. The effector cells are predominantly CD8$^+$ cells, which are phenotypically and functionally identical to the CTLs responsible for killing virus-infected or allogenic cells. Although CD4$^+$ helper T cells are not generally cytotoxic to tumors, thay may provide cytokines for effective CTL development.

CD4$^+$ T cells express surface markers CD25 and FOXP3 transcriptional factors, are recruited by CCR4 and CCR7 chemokines, secrete IL-10 and TGF-β involved in immunosuppression and inhibit inflammation in the tumor microenvironment (Candido and Hagemann 2013). CD4$^+$ TH2 cells secrete IL-4 and stimulate the alternative M2-like activation of TAMs, which entails immunosuppressive, tissue-remodeling, and pro-angiogenic functions (Biswas and Mantovani 2010; De Nardo et al. 2009). IFNγ secreted by CD4$^+$ TH1 cells or CD8$^+$ cytotoxic T cells may stimulate TAMs to up-regulate angiostatic cytokines CXCL9, CXCL10 and CXCL11 (Biswas and Mantovani 2010; Baer et al. 2016).

T cells stimulate angiogenesis synthesizing FGF-2 and heparin-binding epidermal-like growth factor (HB-EGF) (Blotnick et al. 1994). Blockade of VEGF/VEGFR-2 pathway in tumor-bearing mice improves the infiltration of adopetively transferred T cells in the tumor (Shrimali et al. 2010).

NK cells originally were identified in the blood and other lymphoid organs of humans and experimental animals as cells capable of killing a variety of cell types, including tumor-derived cell lines and virus-infected cells. NK cells comprise 10–15% of peripheral blood lymphocytes, and express low amounts of CD56 and high amounts of CD16. Functional NK cells can be detected in the human fetal liver as early as 9–10 weeks of gestation. NK cells are derived from the bone marrow and appear as large lymphocytes with numerous azurophilic cytoplasmatic granules, because of which they are sometimes called large granular lymphocytes. By phenotype, NK cells are neither T nor B cells. NK cells have not phagocytic anctivity and their mediated killing uses the same mechanisms employed in CTL-mediated killing.

The possibility that NK cells provide a link between innate and adaptive immunity is suggested by the observation that NK cells are the major effector cells of the so-called Antibody-Dependent Cell-mediated cytoxicity (ADCC), a function that is also shared by monocyte/macrophages and granulocytes.

In response to high lelels of IL-2, NK cells differentiate into lymphokine-activated killer (LAK) cells. LAK cells exhibit a markedly enhanced capacity to lyse tumor cells and have been used in adoptive immunotherapy of tumors. The incidence of tumors in different strains of imbred mice correlates inversely with the functional capacity of NK cells in these mice. T-cell deficient nude mice have normal or elevated number of NK cells and they do not have a high incidence of spontaneous tumors.

NK cells provide surveillance against tumor cells and virus infected cells (Hayahawa and Smyth 2006). In fact, a higher incidence of lymphoproliferative disorders has been demonstrated in patients with Chidiak-Hagashi syndrome, which have profound deficits in NK activity, and in patients with X-linked lymphoproliferative diseases, NK activity s deficient as well (Sullivan et al. 1980). NK cells often are decreased in pathological conditions, including cancer and AIDS (Trinchieri 1989).

In mice, NK cells have been found essential for the initiation of pregnancy-associated spiral arterial modification through their production of IFN-γ and VEGF. VEGF provides not only a potent pro-angiogenic stimulus but works as an important stem cell survival factor with ability to recruit cells into the hypoxic environments (Carmeliet and Tessier-Lavigne 2005). Thus, it might act as endothelial tip cell guidance towards hypoxic endometrium not only in the endometrial/decidual environment occupied by the trophoblasts but also in the necrotic milieu that occurs during endometrial destruction in the menstrual cycle. Moreover, uterine NK cells contribute to the physiological vascular remodeling in the uterus during the secretory phase of menstrual cycle as well as during pregnancy (Zhang et al. 2011).

A pro-tumorigenic phenotype of cancer infiltrating NK cells has been demonstrated due to their ability to relase angiogenic factors and immunosuppressive cytokines (Bruno et al. 2014).

Experimental work suggests that NK cells are required mediators of angiogenesis inhibition by IL-12, and that NK cell cytotoxicity of endothelial cells is a potential mechanism by which IL-12 can suppress neovascularization (Yao et al. 1999). IL-12 receptors indeed are present primarily on NK cells and T cells (Trinchieri 1993). IL-12-activated lymphocytes influence inhibition of tumor growth and function as an anti-vascular agent, by releasing higher level of IFN-γ and down-modulating VEGF (Cavallo et al. 2001).

The genetic inactivation of Stat5, which is required for NK-cell mediated immunosurveillance, upregulates VEGF-A in NK cells and enhanves angiogenesis in a mouse lymphoma models (Gotthardt et al. 2016).

7.4.1 Lymphocytes, Angiogenesis and Inflammation

Lymphocytes have important pro-angiogenic functions in the course of pregnancy. In particular, NK cells are the most abundant leukocytes in preimplantation endometrium, accumulate and actively proliferate in the endometrium of murine, porcine and human developing placenta (Leonard et al. 2006). In non small cell lung cancer, NK cells synthesize higher VEGF and placental growth factor (PlGF) as compared to controls (Bruno et al. 2013).

Lymphocytes are essential for the airway remodeling. Studies have been performed in mice chronically infected with *Mycoplasma pneumoniae*. Mice lacking B cells expressed a great reduction of angiogenesis when infected with this microorganism (Aurora et al. 2005). The humoral response, indeed, causes deposition of immune complexes on the airway wall, followed by recruitment of inflammatory cells at sites of infected airways which, in turn, are responsible for local production of remodeling factors. In asthma, key cells of allergy such as mast cells, produce significant amounts of IL-1 that contributes to lymphocyte infiltration (Bochner et al. 1990) and IL-4, essential for the triggering of TH2 lymphocytes that themselves produce IL-4 to initiate inflammatory cell accumulation and B lymphocytes immunoglobulin class switching to IgE (Bradding et al. 1993).

VEGF, HIF-1α, TNF-α, IL-8 and Angs are the main players responsible for the strong vessel formation in psoriasis. The proangiogenic milieu in the skin seems to result from a proinflammatory immune response initiated by T helper cells. Several small molecules used for systemic therapy of psoriasis have been shown to provide not only immune regulatory effects but also influence endothelial cell biology. Thus, direct targeting of angiogenesis may not only help to understand psoriasis pathogenesis but also to develop new strategies to treat psoriasis with therapeutics that halt the angiogenesis required for the inflammatory disease. Trangenic mice expressing VEGF under the keratin 14 promoter develop a psoriasis-like inflammation characterized by increased angiogenesis, acanthosis, and immune cell infiltration. It has also been shown that application of 12-O-tetradecanoylphorbol-13-acetate (TPA) in these mice induces a severe and long-lasting skin inflammation with a Th17 cell signature.

Lymphocytes isolated from inflamed ears show a significantly higher number of activated T cells, in contrast to the primarily naive lymphocytes isolated from blood. In addition, there is an increase in regulatory T cells (CD 4+, CD25-, CD127 -/low) within the skin. Interestingly, CD4 depletion results in augmented ear thickness and proinflammatory cytokine levels, indicating that CD4+ T cells have a suppressive rather than a proinflammatory function in this model. Subsequently, sorted regulatory CD4+ CD25+ T cells are transferred to naive K14/VEGF transgenic mice before TPA challenge. CD4+ CD25+ T-cell transfer significantly reduces ear thickness and proinflammatory cytokine production compared to controls, indicating that a persistent skin inflammation with similarities to psoriasis can be controlled by a single injection of few regulatory T cells (Teige et al. 2009).

Lymphocytes may cooperate to the generation of an antiangiogenic microenvironment that is essential for causing regression of the tumor mass. For instance, TH cells and cytotoxic T cells are needed to mediate the anti-angiogenic effect of IL-12 (Strasly et al. 2001).

7.5 Dendritic Cells

Dendritic cells are bone marrow, hematopoietic-derived, professional antigen-presenting cells, able to induce both primary and secondary T- and B-cell responses as well as immune tolerance (Banchereau et al. 2000), and participate in the regulation of the inflammatory reaction through the release of cytokines and chemokines (Banchereau and Steinman 1998).

Dendritic cell development can be broken down into five steps: proliferating progenitors, nonproliferating precursors, immature dendritic cells, mature dendritic cells, and death by apoptosis. Mature dendritic cells lack nonspecific esterase, abundant acid phosphatases and myeloperoxidase and lysozime. CD14 is absent and Fc receptors are scarce. The mature dendritic cells are noadherent to glass or plastic and are poorly or not all pahgocytic.

There are two types of dendritic cells, interdigitating and follicular dendritic cells. Interdigitating cells are present in the interstitium of most organs, are abundant in T cell-rich areas of lymph nodes and spleen, and are scattered throughout the epidermis, where they are called Langerhans cells. Interdigitating cells are not phagocytic cells bur carries antigen from the periphery to present it to T cells in the paracortex of the lymph nodes. Interdigitating cells carry on their surface, the Ia antigen of the major histocompatibility complex, which is able to cluster T cells to facilitate their development as well their sorting and homing.

The follicular cells are present in the germinal centers of lymphoid follicles in the lymph nodes, and mucosa-associated lymphoid tissues. Follicular cells are not phagocytic but retain antigens for prolonged periods, captured in the form of immune complexes. They have implicated in the generation of memory lymphocytes and the maintenance of antibody production.

Dendritic cells are seeded in all tissues and provide an essential link between the innate and adaptive immune responses and when compared with other antigen-presenting cells, such as macrophages, they are extremely efficient. Dendritic cells are present within the stroma of different tumors, including stomach, colon, prostate, kidney, thyroid, breast, and melanoma. Dendritic cells with immunosuppressive regulatory activity are found in different advanced solid tumors (Veglia and Gabrilovich 2017).

Dendritic cells express both pro- and anti angiogenic mediators when exposed to different combinations of cytokines and microbial stimuli and both positive and negative mediators of the angiogenic process can affect the biology of dendritic cells (Fig. 7.9), which express both VEGFR-1 and VEGFR-2 (Mimura et al. 2006). Furthermore, expression of the VEGF co-receptor neuropilin-1 is induced during *in vitro* differentiation of monocytes into dendritic cells (Bourbie-Vaudaine et al. 2006).

Riboldi et al. (2005) reported that dendritic cells can be activated to an angiogenesis-promoting phenotype. They demonstrated that alternative activation of dendritic cells by anti-inflammatory molecules, such as calcitriol, prostaglandin E_2 (PGE_2) or IL-10 prompts them to secrete VEGF and inhibit their secretion of IL-12, a potent antiangiogenic molecule that is secreted by classical activated dendritic cells.

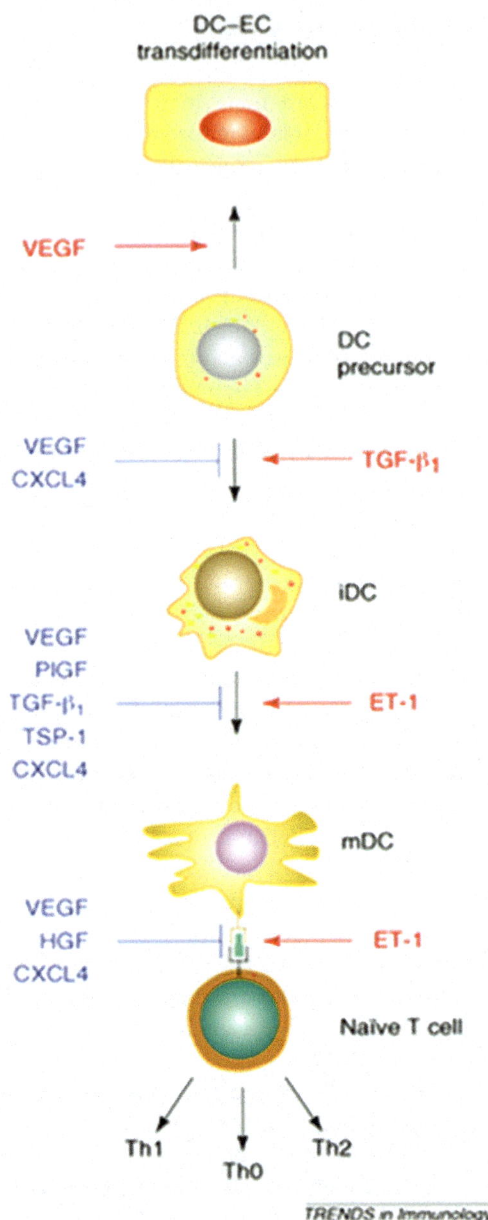

Fig. 7.9 Effect of pro- and anti-angiogenic mediators on dendritic cells (DCs). Various pro- and anti-angiogenic factors inhibit (in blue) the differentiation of myeloid DC precursors in immature dendritic cells (iDCs) and the functional maturation of iDCs to mature DCs (mDCs). Also, they modulate the antigen-presenting function and polarization of mDCs. Others promote DC maturation and function (ET-1) or Langerhans DC differentiation (TGF-β1). Finally, VEGF promotes the transdifferentiation of DC precursors into endothelial-like cells. ET-1, endothelin-1; HGF, hepatocyte growth factor; PlGF, placental growth factor; TGF, transforming growth factor; TSP-1, thrombospondin-1 (Reproduced from Sozzani et al. 2007)

Incubation of tumor associated dendritic cells with VEGF and oncostatin M led to their transdifferentiation in endothelial cells (Gottfried et al. 2007). These cells express classical endothelial cell markers, including von willebrand factor and VE-cadherin and are able to form vascular-like tubes on Matrigel.

Tumor-associated dendritic cells release pro-angiogenic cytokines, including TNFα, CXCL8 and osteopontin (Curiel et al. 2004; Feijoo et al. 2005; Konno et al. 2006). Immature dendritic cells can increase the expression of VEGF and CXCL8 under hypoxic conditions (Ricciardi et al. 2008).

7.6 Mast Cells

Mast cells are bone marrow-derived tissue-homing leukocytes, which were first described by Paul Ehrlich in 1878. They are highly versatile cells playing an important role in large spectrum of biological settings, including inflammation, angiogenesis, tissue repair, tissue remodeling and cancer.

Mast cells are involved in innate immunity through the release of TNF-α, IL-1, Il-4, and IL-6. Moreover, mast cells express major histocompatibility class II (MHC II) molecule and its co-stimulatory molecule, which activate adaptive T- and B-cell response. Mast cells express Toll-like receptors (TLRs), a type of patterns recognition receptor (PRR), which recognize molecules that are shared by pathogens and collectively referred as pathogen-associated molecular patterns (PAMPs). However, the ability of TLRs to stimulate mast cell degranulation, migration and cytokine/chemokine secretion is controversial (Sanding and Bulfone-paus 2013).

Mast cells differ from basophils in the ultrastructure of their cytoplasmic granules, including scroll-like components, crystal-like or particulate substructures, and apparently homogeneous material (Dvorak 1989).

Mast cells produce a large spectrum of pro-angiogenic factors (Fig. 7.10). Human, rat and mouse mast cells release preformed FGF-2 from their secretory granules (Qu et al. 1995, 1998). Human cord blood-derived mast cells release VEGF upon stimulation through FcεRI and c-kit. Both FGF-2 and VEGF have also been identified by immunohistochemistry in mature mast cells in human tissues (Qu et al. 1998; Grutzkau et al. 1998). Human mast cells are a potent source of VEGF in the absence of degranulation through activation of the EP (2) receptor by PGE_2 (Abdel-Majid and Marshall 2004). Following IgE-dependent activation mast cells released several pro-angiogenic mediators stored in their granules, such as VEGF (Boesiger et al. 1998) and FGF-2 (Kanbe et al. 2000), that promote angiogenesis even in the early phase of allergic inflammation. Mast cells can also migrate *in vivo* and *in vitro* in response to VEGF (Detmar et al. 1998; Gruber et al. 1995) and PlGF-1 and express VEGFRs (Fig. 7.11) (Detoraki et al. 2009), suggesting their recruitment to sites of neovascularization during physiological and pathological angiogenesis. Human lung mast cells express VEGF-A, VEGF-B, VEGF-C and VEGF-D at both mRNA and protein level (Detoraki et al. 2009). Moreover, PGE_2 enhanced the expression of VEGF-A, VEGF-B and VEGF-C, whereas an adenosine analog

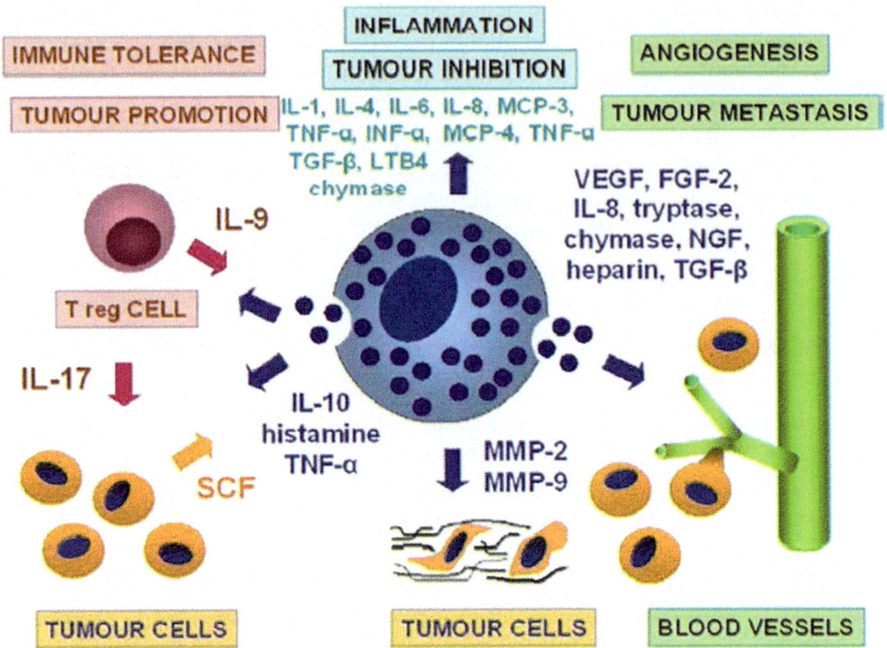

Fig. 7.10 Mast cells attracted in the tumor context by SCF secreted by tumor cells produce several angiogenic factors, such as VEGF, FGF-2, IL-8, tryptase, chymase, NGF, heparin, and TGF-β, as well as matrix metalloproteinases, like MMP-2 and MMP-9, which promote tumor vascularization and tumor invasiveness, respectively. Mast cells may also generate immunosuppression by releasing IL-10, histamine, and TNF-α. Moreover, mast cells infiltrating the tumor stroma favor expansion and activation of regulatory T cells (T reg cells), which, in turn, stimulate immune tolerance and tumor promotion. By contrast, mast cells may promote inflammation, inhibition of tumor cell growth, and tumor cell apoptosis by releasing cytokines such as IL-1, IL-4, IL-6, IL-8, MCP-3, MCP-4, INF-α, TNF-α, TGF-β, LTB4, and chymase (Reproduced from Ribatti and Crivellato 2012)

(5′-(N-ethylcarboxamido) adenosine (NECA)) increased VEGF-A, VEGF-C and VEGF-D expression. Finally, supernatants of PGE$_2$- and NECA-activated human lung mast cells induced angiogenic response in the CAM assay that was inhibited by an anti-VEGF-A antibody (Detoraki et al. 2009).

PGE2 dose-dependently induces primary mast cells to release the pro-angiogenic chemokine monocyte chemoattractant protein-1 (MCP-1) (Nakayama et al. 2006). This release of MCP-1 is complete by 2 hours after PGE2 exposure, reaches levels of MCP-1 at least 15-fold higher than background, and is not accompanied by degranulation or increased MCP-1 gene expression. By immunoelectron microscopy, MCP-1 is detected within mast cells at a cytoplasmic location distinct from the secretory granules. Dexamethasone and cyclosporine A inhibit PGE2-induced MCP-1 secretion by approximately 60%. Agonists of PGE2 receptor subtypes revealed that the EP1 and EP3 receptors can independently mediate MCP-1 release from mast cells. These observations identify PGE2-induced MCP-1 release from

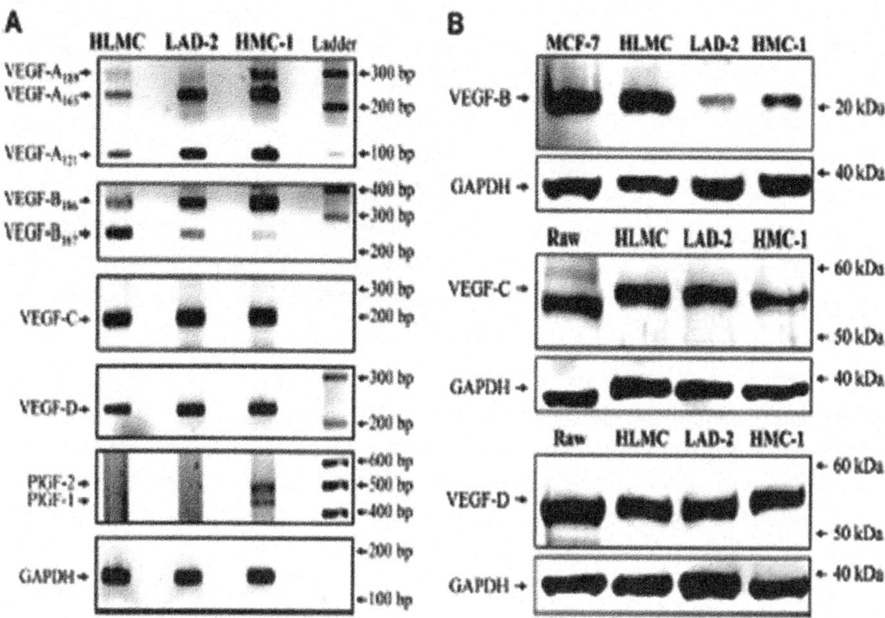

Fig. 7.11 Expression of VEGFs in human mast cells. A, VEGF-A, VEGF-B, VEGF-C, VEGF-D and PlGF RT-PCR amplification products from human lung mast cells (HLMCs), LAD-2 cells, and HMC-1 cells. B, Immunoblot with anti–VEGF-B, anti–VEGF-C, anti–VEGF-D, and anti–GAPDH antibodies of HLMC, LAD-2, and HMC-1 lysates. MCF-7 and RAW 264.7 (Raw) cells were used as positive controls. (Reproduced from Detoraki et al. 2009)

mast cells as a pathway underlying inflammation-associated angiogenesis and extend current understanding of the activities of PGE2.

Granulated mast cells and their granules, but not degranulated mast cells, are able indeed to stimulate an intense angiogenic reaction in the CAM assay. This angiogenic activity is partly inhibited by anti-FGF-2 and anti-VEGF antibodies, suggesting that these cytokines are involved in the angiogenic reaction (Ribatti et al. 2001). Intraperitoneal injection of the degranulating compound 48/80 causes a strong angiogenic response in the rat mesentery window angiogenic assay and in mice (Norrby ct al. 1986, 1989).

Mast cells contain MMPs (HMC-1 constitutively express MMP-9 mRNA and secrete active form of MMP-9 following PMA activation) and tissue inhibitors of metalloproteinases (TIMPs), (Tanaka et al. 2001; Koskivirta et al. 2006) which intervene in regulation of extracellular matrix degradation, allowing release of angiogenic factors.

Mast cells store large amounts of preformed active serine proteases, such as tryptase and chymase, in their secretory granules (Metcalfe et al. 1997). Tryptase stimulates the proliferation of endothelial cells, promotes vascular tube formation in culture and also degrades connective tissue matrix to provide space for neovascular growth (Ribatti and Ranieri 2015). Tryptase also acts indirectly by activating latent

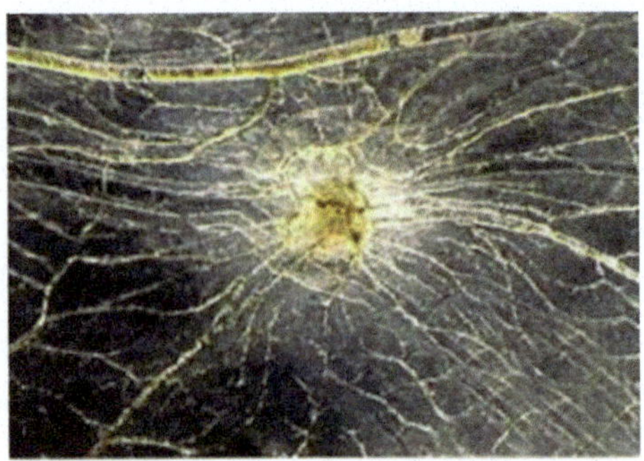

Fig. 7.12 Tryptase is angiogenic in vivo in the CAM assay. Macroscopic picture of CAMs at day 12 of incubation treated with tryptase. Note the presence of numerous blood vessels converging toward the implant (Modified from Ribatti et al. 2011)

MMPs and plasminogen activator (PA), which in turn degrade the extracellular connective tissue with consequent release of VEGF or FGF-2 from their matrix-bound state (Blair et al. 1997), and is angiogenic in the CAM assay (Fig. 7.12) (Ribatti et al. 2011). Mast cell-derived chymase degrades extracellular matrix components and therefore matrix-bound VEGF could be potentially released. The expression of chymase and tryptase correlates with mast cell maturation and angiogenesis during tumor progression in chemically induced tumor growth in BALB/c mouse (de Souza et al. 2012).

Histamine and heparin stimulated proliferation of endothelial cells induced the formation of new blood vessels in the CAM-assay (Ribatti et al. 1987; Sorbo et al. 1994). Histamine stimulates new vessel formation by acting through both H1 and H2 receptors (Sorbo et al. 1994). In an in vivo system of induced subcutaneous granuloma, histamine induced angiogenesis by up-regulating VEGF. The effect was delayed when the subcutaneous granuloma was induced in mice lacking histamine (L-histidine decarboxylase knock out mice). Histamine modulates tumor growth through H1 and H2 receptors (Fitzsimons et al. 1997). H1 receptor antagonists significantly improved overall survival rates and suppressed tumor growth as well as the infiltration of mast cells and VEGF levels through the inhibition of HIF-1α expression in B16F10 melanoma-bearing mice (Jeong et al. 2013).

Heparin may act directly on blood vessels or indirectly by inducing release of FGF-2 from the extracellular storage site. Mast cell-derived heparin stimulates capillary endothelial migration and proliferation in vitro. In in vivo experiments, the s.c. injection of commercial standard heparin (mean 15 kD) and high molecular weight heparin (mean 22 kD) stimulates angiogenesis, wheras low molecular weight heparin (mean 2.5 amd 5.0 kD) inhibits it. These different effects suggest that the molecular size and tertiary structure of heparin may influence angiogenesis. Heparin could facilitate tumor vascularization not only by a direct pro-angiogenic effect but also through its anti-clotting effect (Theoharides and Conti 2004).

Other cytokines produced by mast cells, including IL-8 (Moller et al. 1993), TNF-α (Walsh et al. 1991), TGF-β, NGF (Nilsson et al. 1997) and urokinase-type PA are involved in normal and tumor-associated angiogenesis (Aoki et al. 2003).

Although some evidence suggest that these cells can promote tumorigenesis and tumor progression, there are some clinical data as well as experimental tumor models in which mast cells seems to have functions that favor the host (Ribatti and Crivellato 2009). Mast cells exert immunosuppression releasing TNF-α and IL-10, which are essential in promoting the immune tolerance mediated by regulatory T (Treg) cells, and stimulate immune tolerance and tumor promotion (Ullrich et al. 2007; Grimbaldeston et al. 2007). Mast cells promote inflammation, inhibition of tumor cell growth, and tumor cell apoptosis by releasing cytokines, such as interleukin IL-1, IL-4, IL-6, IL-8, monocyte chemotactic protein-3 and -4 (MCP-3 and MCP-4), TGF-β, and chymase. Chondrotin sulphate may inhibit tumor cells diffusion and tryptase causes both tumor cell disruption and inflammation through activation of protease-activated receptors (PAR-1 and -2) (Ribatti and Crivellato 2012).

Mast cell-deficient W/Wv mice exhibit a decreased rate of tumor angiogenesis (Starkey et al. 1988). Development of squamous cell carcinoma in a human papilloma virus (HPV) 16 infected transgenic mouse model of epithelia carcinogenesis provided experimental support for the early participation of mast cells in tumor growth and angiogenesis (Coussens et al. 1999, 2000). Mast cells infiltrated hyperplasia, dysplasias, and the invasive front of carcinomas, but not the core of tumors. Accumulation occurred proximal to developing capillaries and the stroma surrounding the advancing tumor mass (Coussens et al. 1999). Infiltration of mast cells and activation of MMP-9 coincided with the angiogenic switch in premalignant lesions through the release of pro-angiogenic molecules from the extracellular matrix. Remarkably, premalignant angiogenesis was abrogated in a mast cell-deficient HPV 16 transgenic mouse indicating that neoplastic progression in this model involved infiltration of mast cells in the skin (Coussens et al. 1999, 2000). By using the same in vivo transgenic mouse model, it has been demonstrated that genetic elimination of mature T and B lymphocytes, limits neoplastic progression (de Visser et al. 2005; Andreu et al. 2010). Moreover, in prostate tumors derived from both tumor transgenic adenocarcinoma of the mouse prostate (TRAMP) mice and human patients, mast cells promote well-differentiated adenocarcinoma growth (Pittoni et al. 2011).

Within the developing tumor environment, mast cells do not act alone. As tumor growth progresses, mast cells recruit eosinophils and neutrophils and activate T and B cell immune responses (Kinet 2007).

An increased number of mast cells has indeed been reported in angiogenesis associated with vascular neoplasms, like haemangioma and haemangioblastoma (Glowacki and Mulliken 1982), as well as a number of solid and haematopoietic tumors. Mast cell density correlates with angiogenesis and poor tumor outcome. Association between mast cells and new vessel formation has been reported in breast cancer (Hartveit 1981; Bowrey et al. 2000), gastric cancer (Fig. 7.13) (Yano et al. 1999; Ribatti et al. 2010), colorectal cancer (Lachter et al. 1995) and uterine cervix cancer (Graham and Graham 1966). Tryptase-positive mast cells increase in number and vascularization increases in a linear fashion from dysplasia to invasive cancer of the uterine cervix (Benitez-Bribiesca et al. 2001; Ribatti et al. 2005). An association of VEGF and mast cells with angiogenesis has been demonstrated in laryngeal carcinoma (Sawatsubashi et al. 2000) and in small lung carcinoma, where

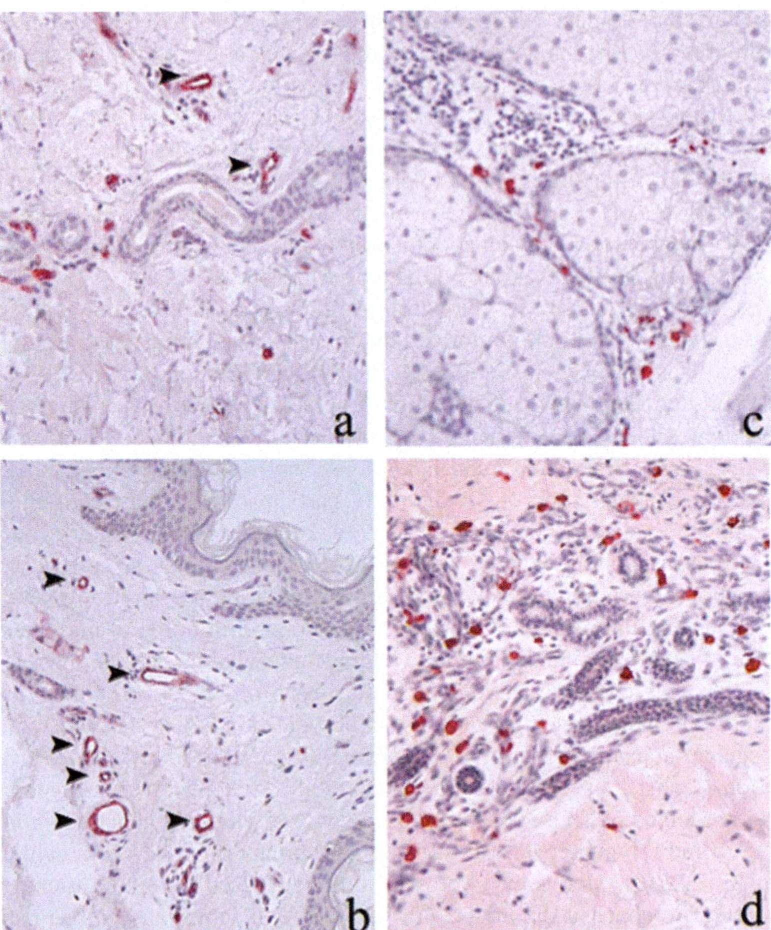

Fig. 7.13 Histological sections of human advanced primary melanomas stained with factor VIII for microvessels (**a,b**) and withm tryptase for mast cells (**c,d**) from patients with good (**a,c**) and poor prognosis (**b,d**) subgroup. Note the higher density of microvessels with an appreciable lumen (arrowheads) and of mast cells (red stained) in the poor prognosis patient (Reproduced from Ribatti et al. 2003a)

most intratumoral mast cells express VEGF (Imada et al. 2000; Takanami et al. 2000; Tomita et al. 2000). Mast cell accumulation has also been noted around invasive melanoma (Reed et al. 2006; Dvorak et al. 1980). In melanoma, mast cell accumulation was correlated with increased neovascularization, mast cell expression of VEGF (Toth-Jakatics et al. 2000) and FGF-2 (Ribatti et al. 2003a), tumor aggressiveness and poor prognosis. Indeed, a prognostic significance has been attributed to mast cells and microvascular density in melanoma (Fig. 7.14) (Ribatti et al. 2003b), and in squanous cell cancer of the oesophagus (Elpek et al. 2001) and squa-

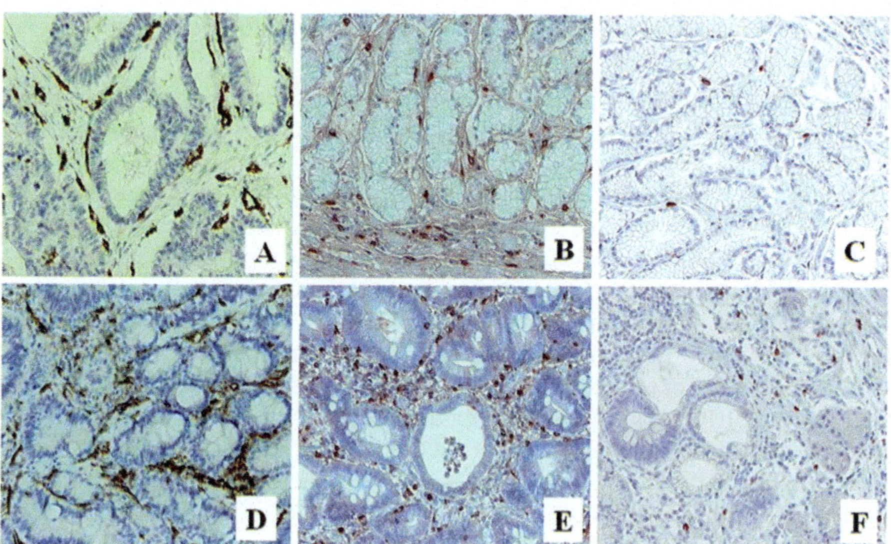

Fig. 7.14 Immunohistochemical staining for CD31, tryptase and chymase in stage II (**a–c**) and stage IV (**d–f**) human gastric cancer. In (**a, d**) endothelial cells immunoreactive for CD31, in (**b, e**) tryptase-positive mast cells; in (**c, f**) chymase-positive mast cells. Blood vessels and mast cells are distributed around the gastric glands. The number of blood vessels and mast cells is higher in stage IV as compared with stage II (Reproduced from Ribatti et al. 2010)

mous cell carcinoma of the lip (Rojas et al. 2005). Data on mast cells and metastasis have been scant and poor.

Mast cell density, new vessel rate and clinical prognosis have correlate in haematological tumors. In benign lymphadenopathies and B cell non-Hodgkin's lymphomas, angiogenesis correlates with total and tryptase-positive mast cell counts, and both increase in step with the increase with malignancy grades (Ribatti et al. 1998, 2000). In non-Hodgkin's lymphomas, a correlation has been found between vessel count and the number of mast cells and VEGF-expressing cells (Fukushima et al. 2001). In the bone marrow of patients with inactive and active multiple myeloma as well as those with monoclonal gammopathies of undetermined significance, angiogenesis highly correlates with mast cell counts (Ribatti et al. 1999). A similar pattern of correlation between bone marrow microvessel count, total and tryptase-positive mast cell density and tumor progression has been found in patients with myelodysplastic syndrome (Ribatti et al. 2002) and B cell chronic lymphocytic leukemia (Ribatti et al. 2003c). In the early stages of B cell chronic lymphocytic leukemia, the density of tryptase-positive mast cells in the bone marrow predicts the outcome of the disease (Molica et al. 2003).

7.6.1   *Mast Cells, Angiogenesis, and Chronic Inflammation*

Mast cells are common components of inflammatory infiltrates and exert basic functions in the cross-talk between immunological, inflammatory and reparative tissue reactions (Metcalfe et al. 1997).

Myocardial infarction is associated with an acute inflammatory response, leading to replacement of injured cardiomyocytes with granulation tissue (Ren et al. 2003). Myocardial necrosis is associated with complement activation and free radical generation, triggering a cytokine cascade and chemokine upregulation. IL-8 and C5a are released in the ischemic myocardium, and may have a crucial role in neutrophil recruitment. Extravasated neutrophils may induce potent cytotoxic effects through the release of proteolytic enzymes and the adhesion with intercellular adhesion molecule (ICAM)-1 expressing cardiomyocytes. MCP-1 is induced in the infarcted area and may regulate mononuclear cell recruitment. Accumulation of monocyte-derived macrophages, and mast cells may increase expression of growth factors inducing angiogenesis and fibroblast accumulation in the infarct. In addition, expression of cytokines inhibiting the inflammatory response, such as IL-10 may suppress injury. MMPs and their inhibitors regulate extracellular matrix deposition and play an important role in mediating ventricular remodeling. Mast cells are actively involved in postinfarction inflammation by releasing histamine and TNF-α, triggering a cytokine cascade. During the proliferative phase of healing, mast cells accumulate in the infarct and may regulate fibrous tissue deposition and angiogenesis by releasing growth factors, angiogenic mediators, and proteases. In the healing infarct, mast cells are associated with other cell types that are important for granulation tissue formation. Inflammatory mediators may induce recruitment of blood-derived primitive stem cells in the healing infarct, which may differentiate into endothelial cells and even lead to limited myocardial regeneration.

Mast cells have been implied in the neovascularization associated with rosacea. Indeed, angiogenesis seems to play an important role in the pathogenesis especially of the more severe clinical form of rosacea. Mast cells seem to participate in evolution to disease chronicity by contributing to inflammation, angiogenesis and tissue fibrosis (Aroni et al. 2007).

Atopic dermatitis skin lesions are characterized by inflammatory changes and epithelial hyperplasia requiring angiogenesis. Mast cells may participate in this process via bidirectional secretion of tissue-damaging enzymes and pro-angiogenic factors. It has been shown that mast cells are abundantly localized in the papillary dermis and migrate through the basal lamina into the epidermis of atopic dermatitis lesions (Groneberg et al. 2005). Approximately 80% are chymase positive. A high number of mast cells express c-kit. Most papillary and epidermal mast cells localize close to endothelial cells. Vascular expression of endoglin (CD105) demonstrates neoangiogenic processes. Mast cells stimulation leads to the expression of proangiogenic factors and tissue-damaging factors such MMPs. These data suggest that in atopic dermatitis, mast cells close to papillary vessels and within the epidermis may be implicated in stimulation of neoangiogenesis.

Mast cells are involved in the pathogenesis of rheumatoid arthritis (Yamada et al. 1998). Mast cells reside in connective tissues and in synovial tissue of joints. They produce an array of proinflammatory mediators, tissue destructive proteases, and cytokines, most prominently TNF-α, which is one of the key cytokines in the pathogenesis of rheumatoid arthritis (Eklund 2007).

Mast cells may also participate in the development of secondary or amyloid A amyloidosis, as the partial degradation of the serum amyloid A protein by mast cells leads to the generation of a highly amyloidogenic N-terminal fragment of serum amyloid A. Mast cells may contribute to the pathogenesis of connective tissue diseases, scleroderma, vasculitic syndromes, and systemic lupus erythematosus. Inhibition of the most important growth factor receptor of human mast cells, c-Kit, by the selective tyrosine kinase inhibitor imatinib mesylate, induces apoptosis of synovial tissue mast cells. As mast cells are long-lived cells, induction of their apoptosis could be a feasible approach to inhibit their functions.

Mast cells have been implicated in the vascular inflammation leading to aneurism formation. Abdominal aortic aneurysm is histologically characterized by medial degeneration and various degrees of chronic adventitial inflammation, although the mechanisms for progression of aneurysm are poorly understood. The number of mast cells was found to increase in the outer media or adventitia of human abdominal aortic aneurysm, showing a positive correlation between the cell number and the aneurism diameter (Tsuruda et al. 2008). Aneurysmal dilatation of the aorta was seen in the control rats following periaortic application of calcium chloride (CaCl2) treatment but not in the mast cell-deficient mutant Ws/Ws rats. The aneurism formation was accompanied by accumulation of mast cells, T lymphocytes and by activated MMP-9, reduced elastin levels and augmented angiogenesis in the aortic tissue, but these changes were much less in the Ws/Ws rats than in the controls. Similarly, mast cells accumulated and activated at the adventitia of aneurysmal aorta in the apolipoprotein E-deficient mice. The pharmacological intervention with the tranilast, an inhibitor of mast cell degranulation, attenuated aneurism development in these rodent models. In the cell culture experiment, mast cells directly augmented MMP-9 activity produced by the monocyte/macrophage. These data suggest that adventitial mast cells play a critical role in the progression of abdominal aortic aneurysm.

7.6.2   Therapeutic Strategies

Mast cells might act as a new target for the adjuvant treatment of tumors through the selective inhibition of angiogenesis, tissue remodeling and tumor promoting molecules, allowing the secretion of cytotoxic cytokines and preventing mast cell mediated immune-suppression. Pre-clinical studies using anti-cKIT antibodies (Huang et al. 2008), anti-TNF-α antibodies (Gounaris et al. 2007), or the mast cells stabilizer disodium cromoglycate (cromolyn) (Soucek et al. 2007) in mouse models have demonstrated promising results.

Histamine receptor antagonists have anti-angiogenic properties in vitro and in vivo (De Luisi et al. 2009; Kubecova et al. 2011). Inhaled corticosteroids have beneficial effects on angiogenesis, permeability and vessel dilatation mediated by reducing the ratio of VEGF/Ang-2 and modulating the balance of VEGF and endostatin, inhibiting the production of CXCL-8, GM-CSF, TNF, and MMPs (Chetta et al. 2007). Treatment with nonsteroidal anti-inflammatory drugs reduces the incidence of colorectal cancer (Kochne and Dubois 2004).

7.7   Eosinophils

Peripheral blood and tissue eosinophils are derived from CD34-positive myelocytic progenitors found in the bone marrow and inflamed tissues. Eosinophils contain four granule types: primary granules, secondary specific granules (or crystalloid granules), small granules, and secretory vesicles. The eosinophil is characterized by large crystalloid granules, as shown in light microscopy by their bright red staining properties with eosin. At ultrastructural level, the crystalloid granules contain electron-dense crystalline cores surrounded by an electron-lucent granule matrix. The major basic protein (MBP), toxic for some helminths, is contained in the crystalloid. Primary granules contain Charcot-Leyden crystals, observed in fluids in association with eosinophilic inflammatory reactions. Human eosinophils produce over 25 different cytokines, chemokines, and growth factors, involved in the regulation of different immune responses (Table 7.6). Other granule-stored proteins include different enzymes involved in inflammation, such as phosphatase, collagenase, MMPs, histaminases, catalase, and phospholypase D.

Eosinophilia accompanies different pathological conditions, including helmintic parasites, atopic allergic diseases, seasonal and perennial rhinitis, atopic dermatitis, and asthma. Moreover, eosinophilia is associated to a variety of lymphoid and solid tumors, particularly Hodgkin lymphoma. Eosinophils are recruited to tumors by

Table 7.6 Cytokines, chemokines and growth factors produced by human eosinophils

Interleukins (IL)
IL-1α, IL-2, IL-3, IL-4, IL-5, IL-6, IL-9, IL-10, IL-11, IL-12, IL-13, IL-16, Leukemia inhibitory factor (LIF)
Interferon gamma
Tumor necrosis factor
Granulocyte-Mancrophage Colony Stimulating Factor
Chemokines
Eotaxin, IL-8, MIP-1α, MCP-1, MCP-3, MCP-4, RANTES
Growth factors
EGF, NGF, PDGF-B, TGF-α, TGF-β1

CC-chemokine ligand 11 (CCL11, also known as eotaxin) through CC-chemokine receptor 3 (CCR3) and localize to hypoxic tumor areas (Cormier et al. 2006).

Eosinophils are pro-angiogenic through the production of an array of cytokines and growth factors, such as VEGF, FGF-2, TNFα, GM-CSF, NGF, IL-8 and angiogenin (Horiuchi et al. 1997; Hoshino et al. 2001a; Wong et al. 1990; Kita et al. 1991; Solomon et al. 1998; Yousefi et al. 1995; Hoshino et al. 2001b), and are positively stained for VEGF and FGF-2 in the airways of asthmatic patients (Hoshino et al. 2001a). Eosinophils release VEGF following stimulation with GM-CSF and IL-5 (Hoshino et al. 2001a), both expressed in the tissue and in the bronchoalveolar lavage fluid of patients with allergic asthma. Eosinophils generate VEGF by de novo synthesis and release it (Horiuchi et al. 1997). VEGFR-1 and -2 have been detected on human peripheral blood eosinophils and VEGF induces eosinophil migration and cationic protein release, mainly through VEGFR-1 (Feistritzer et al. 2004). Eosinophils promoted endothelial cells proliferation *in vitro* and induce new vessel formation in the aorta ring and in the CAM assays (Figs. 7.15, 7.16, and 7.17) (Puxeddu et al. 2005a, b). Neutralization of VEGF in eosinophils reduced their angiogenic effects in the CAM by 55% suggesting the important, but not unique role played by this factor in the induction of the angiogenic response. Eosinophils are not the only source of VEGF but they can also be targets for VEGF in allergic inflammation. Eosinophil infiltration could be reduced by administration of an anti-VEGF receptor antibody in a murine model of toluene diisocyanate (TDI)-induced asthma (Lee et al. 2002). Eosinophils are a rich source of preformed MMP-9, and they promote angiogenesis also by acting on matrix degradation.

Eosinophil-derived major basic protein (MBP) induced endothelial cell proliferation and enhanced the pro-mitogenic effect of VEGF, but did not affect VEGF release (Figs. 7.18, and 7.19) (Puxeddu et al. 2009). Moreover, MBP promoted capillarogenesis by endothelial cells seeded on Matrigel, angiogenesis in vivo in the CAM assay, and the pro-angiogenic effect of MBP was not due to its cationic charge since stimulation in the CAM with the synthetic polycation, poly-L-arginine did not induce any angiogenic effect (Puxeddu et al. 2009). Hypoxia increases eosinophil survival, HIF-1α, VEGF, and CXCL8 release (Nissim Ben Efrain et al. 2010).

Eosinophils are blood circulating granulocytes that have an important role both in the development of allergic inflammation and in the pathophysiology of tissue remodeling (Munitz and Levi-Schaffer 2004). They are key cells in the late stages of allergic inflammation. In several conditions such as asthma, rhinitis, vernal keratoconjunctivitis and atopic dermatitis these cells contribute to the perpetuation of inflammatory process and to the development of tissue remodeling.

In the majority of nasal polyps, eosinophils comprise more than 60% of the cell population (Pawankar 2003). An increased production of cytokines/chemokines like GM-CSF, IL-5, RANTES and eotaxin contribute to eosinophil migration and survival. Again, increased expression of VEGF and its upregulation by TGF-β can contribute to the edema and increased angiogenesis in nasal polyps.

Although mouse models of inflammatory skin diseases such as psoriasis and atopic dermatitis fail to completely phenocopy disease in humans, they provide

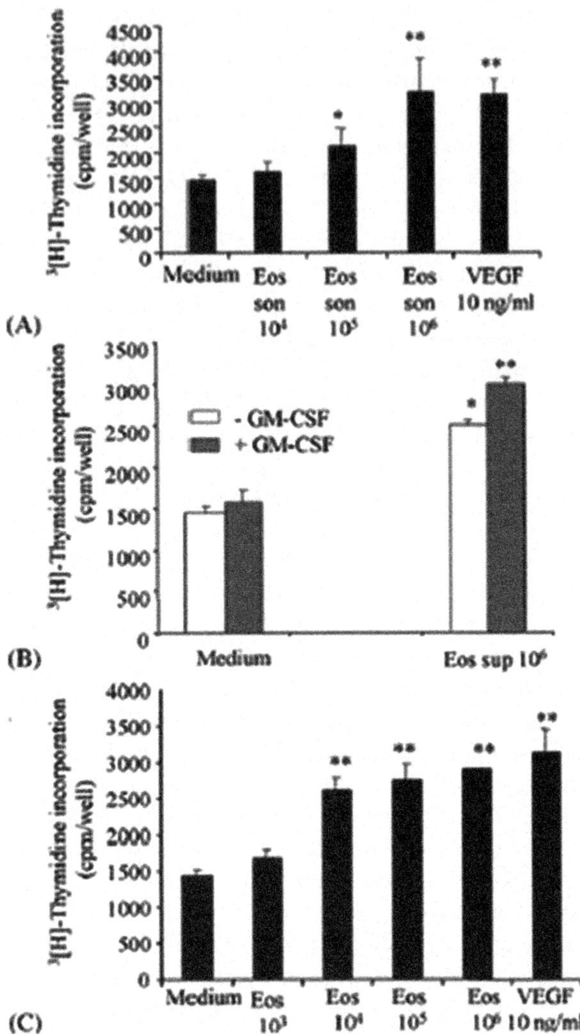

Fig. 7.15 Eosinophils induce endothelial cell proliferation. Subconfluent rat aortic endothelial cells were incubated with eosinophil sonicate (Eos son) (A) or eosinophil supernatants (Eos sup) (B) or co-cultured with freshly isolated eosinophils (Eos) (C) for 24 h. Endothelial cell proliferation was then evaluated by 3(H)-thymidine incorporation. Medium and VEGF were used as negative and positive controls, respectively. (*) $P < 0.05$ and (**) $P < 0.01$ vs. endothelial cells cultured in medium (Reproduced from Puxeddu et al. 2005a, b)

invaluable tools to examine the molecular and cellular mechanisms responsible for the epidermal hyperplasia, inflammation, and excess angiogenesis observed in human disease. Interestingly, treatment of Tie-2 transgenic mice with anti-CD4 antibody resolve aspects of inflammation but did not resolve epidermal hyperplasia, suggesting an important role for eosinophils in mediating the inflammatory skin disease observed in these mice (Voskas et al. 2008). Indeed, there is an increased number of CD3-positive T lymphocytes in the blood and increased infiltration of eosinophils in the skin associated with a deregulated expression of cytokines associated with Th1 and eosinophil immune responses.

The 33-amino acid peptide secretoneurin has been shown to potently and specifically attract eosinophils towards a concentration gradient and acts as an angiogenic

Fig. 7.16 Eosinophils induce rat aorta sprouting. Rat aorta rings grown in collagen gel were incubated with eosinophil sonicate (Eos son) or with medium for 3 days. Microvessel formation was photographed with a stereoscope (**a**) and quantified by direct counting (**b**). $P < 0.05$ and (******) $P < 0.01$ vs. rat aorta rings cultured in medium (Reproduced from Puxeddu et al. 2005a, b)

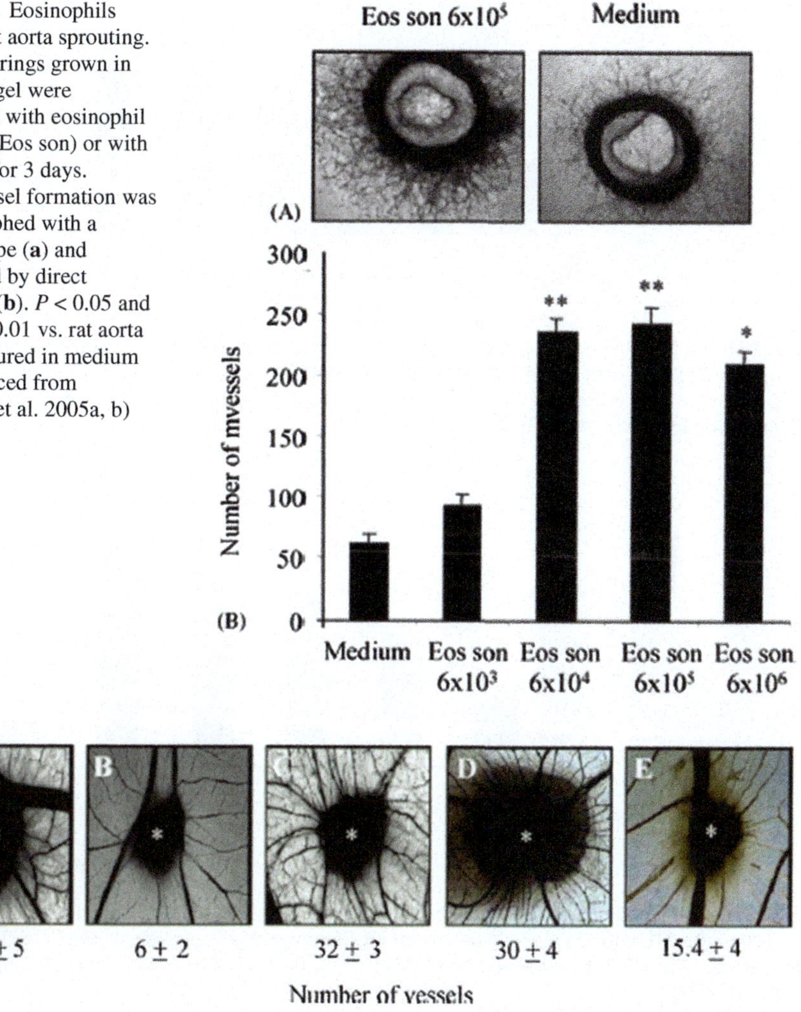

Fig. 7.17 Eosinophils induce an angiogenic response in the chick embryo CAM. Eosinophil sonicate (**a**), medium alone (**b**), cell suspensions of rat mast cells (**c**), VEGF (**d**), or eosinophil sonicate pre-incubated with anti-VEGF neutralizing antibody (**e**) were delivered on the top of the CAM, by using a gelatin sponge implant (asterisk). In **a**, **c** and **d**, gelatin sponges are surrounded by allantoic vessels that develop radially towards the implant in a "spoked-wheel" pattern. In **b**, no vascular reaction is detectable and in E reduced vascular reaction is detectable around the sponge (Reproduced from Puxeddu et al. 2005b)

cytokine comparable in potency to VEGF (Fischer-Colbrie et al. 2005). Thus, secretoneurin contributes to neurogenic inflammation and might play a role in the (hypoxia-driven) induction of neo-vascularisation in ischemic diseases like peripheral or coronary artery disease, diabetic retinopathia, cerebral ischemia or in solid tumors.

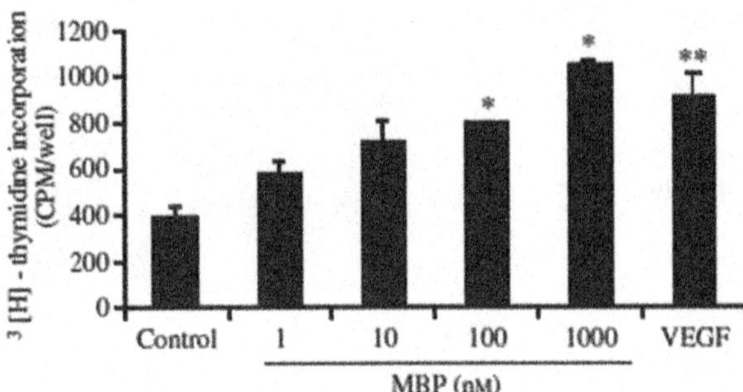

Fig. 7.18 Endothelial cells were incubated with medium alone (control) or with different concentrations of MBP or with VEGF for 24 hours. Endothelial cell proliferation was then evaluated by ^{3}(H)-Thymidine incorporation assay and expressed as CPM/well. *$P < 0.01$, **$P < 0.001$ vs control (Reproduced from Puxeddu et al. 2009)

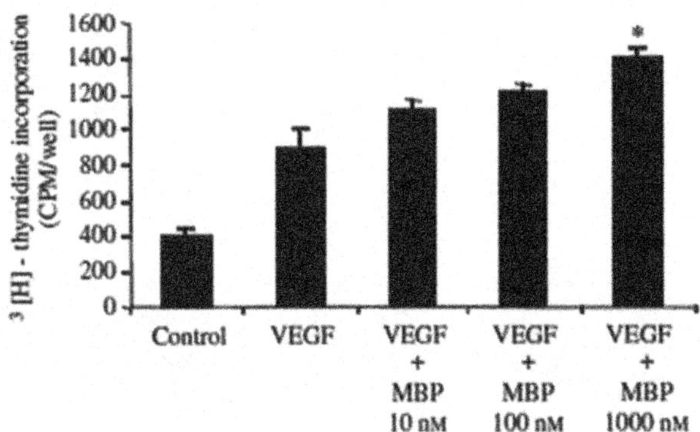

Fig. 7.19 Endothelial cells were incubated with medium alone (control) or with VEGF alone or together with MBP for 24 h. Endothelial cell proliferation was then evaluated by ^{3}(H)-Thymidine incorporation assay and expressed as CPM/well. *$P < 0.01$ vs control (Reproduced from Puxeddu et al. 2009)

7.7.1   Mast Cells and Eosinophils in Angiogenesis During Allergic Diseases

Activated mast cells release mediators that contribute to eosinophil recruitment, activation and survival. For example, rat peritoneal mast cell-derived TNF enhances eosinophil survival by autocrine production of GM-CSF, and mast cell-derived tryptase induces IL-6 and IL-8 release in eosinophils by the mitogen-activated protein kinase (MAPK) and activating protein (AP)-1 pathways. On the other hand, eosinophil-derived mediators can influence mast cell survival and activation. Among them, MBP was found to induce histamine and prostaglandin (PG)D_2 release from human lung and cord blood-derived mast cells through an IgE-independent mechanism. Eosinophils synthesize, store and release important mast cell survival and activating factors such as SCF and NGF. All these evidences indicate that mast cells and eosinophils through their specific preformed mediators can prolong and even intensify allergic inflammation with possible development of tissue damage and consequent remodeling.

Increased vascularity in the airways has been recognized not only in patients with severe asthma, but also in those with mild disease (Li and Wilson 1997; Orsida et al. 1999; Redington et al. 2001). Studies in the airways of asthmatic patients have revealed that the ratio between the level of VEGF and endostatin, pro- and anti-angiogenic mediators respectively, is increased in the sputum of asthmatics in comparison to control subjects (Svensson et al. 1995). Therefore, it seems that an imbalance in favor of pro-angiogenic factors leads to the abnormal growth of new blood vessels in asthma. The submucosa of the airways of asthmatics also exhibits higher VEGF, FGF-2 and angiogenin immunoreactivity than did control subjects (Hoshino et al. 2001a, b), and the expression of VEGF, and VEGFR-1 and VEGFR-2 inversely correlates with airway function (Asai et al. 2002). An increase in FGF-2 levels in the bronchial alveolar lavage (BAL) fluid of atopic asthmatics in comparison to healthy subjects has also been reported (Hoshino et al. 2001a, b). Interestingly, a further increase of FGF-2 in the BAL fluid following acute allergen exposure suggests that the up-regulation of angiogenic mediators may be the result of mast cells degranulation following IgE-dependent activation.

The direct contribution of VEGF in allergic response in asthma has been rproposed by Lee et al. (2004). They generated lung-targeted $VEGF_{165}$ transgenic mice and evaluated the role of VEGF in antigen-induced Th2-mediated inflammation. Over-expression of VEGF induced leukocytes infiltration in the lung, over-production of IL-13, as well as increases in mucus production, collagen deposition and smooth muscle hyperplasia. Interestingly, these mice had an increase in the number of activated dendritic cells, and they developed an exaggerated immune response following respiratory allergen challenge. These results prove that VEGF has direct effects on the immune system and it amplifies a TH2-mediated response in an animal model of experimental asthma.

On the other hand, it has been demonstrated that TH2 cytokines modulate the synthesis and release of VEGF by different inflammatory and structural cells of the airways. For example, in the airway smooth muscle cells IL-4, IL-5 and IL-13 enhanced VEGF production while TH1 cytokines such as IFNγ inhibited their spontaneous and IL-4-, IL-5- or IL-13-induced VEGF release. These results introduce a new concept of how VEGF and the immune system can interact in the allergic airway disorders: TH2 cytokines such as IL-13 induce structural cells to produce VEGF, which, in turn, enhance allergen induced inflammation and consequent remodeling.

Several studies have highlighted the contribution of mast cells in angiogenesis during allergic inflammation. Following IgE-dependent activation mast cells released several pro-angiogenic mediators stored in their granules, such as VEGF and FGF-2, promoting angiogenesis even in the early phase of allergic inflammation. Histamine stimulates new vessel formation by acting through H_1 and H_2 receptors. In an *in vivo* system of induced subcutaneous granuloma, histamine increased angiogenesis by up-regulating the level of VEGF. This effect was delayed when the subcutaneous granuloma was induced in mice lacking histamine. Some experimental evidences indicate that mediators present in allergic inflammation promote the release of pro-angiogenic mediators by mast cells and eosinophils. Eosinophils can release VEGF following stimulation with GM-CSF and IL-5 (Horiuchi and Weller 1997), Moreover IgE-mediated mouse and human mast cell activation is an effective inducer of VEGF production. Interestingly, PGE_2, found to be elevated in allergic asthma, induced human mast cells to release VEGF via activation of the EP2 receptor in the absence of degranulation. Since both mast cells and eosinophils are rich sources of several extracellular matrix-degrading enzymes, we believe that they promote angiogenesis by acting on matrix degradation. HMC-1 constitutively express MMP-9 mRNA and secrete the active form of MMP-9 following PMA activation. Eosinophils were previously found to produce active MMP-9 and more recently we have shown that they express heparanase, an extracellular matrix degrading enzyme that is pre-formed and inhibited by the eosinophil cationic proteins (Temkin et al. 2004). In addition, IL-8, a pro-angiogenic chemokine pre-formed in and newly synthesized by eosinophils, enhances the mRNA levels, as well as active MMP-2 and MMP-9 expression in endothelial cells.

Several cytokines and growth factors involved in allergic inflammation and in remodeling are responsible for increasing the basal level of VEGF in fibroblasts, smooth muscle cells and keratinocytes. Bradykinin, IL-1α, IL-5, IL-13 and TGF-β are potent inducers of VEGF in airway smooth muscle cells, and TGF-β together with IL-4 and IL-13 enhances the synthesis of VEGF in bronchial fibroblasts (Richter et al. 2001). VEGF is a potent chemoattractant for leukocytes in experimental asthma (Lee et al. 2004) and induces migration of mononuclear cells across an endothelial cell monolayer *in vitro*. Eosinophil infiltration could be reduced by administration of anti-VEGF receptor antibodies in a murine model of toluene diisocyanate (TDI)-induced asthma (Lee et al. 2002). A possible explanation for this down-regulatory effect comes from recent *in vitro* studies. VEGFR-1 and -2 have been detected on human peripheral blood eosinophils and VEGF induces eosinophil migration and ECP release, mainly through VEGFR-1 (Feistritzer et al. 2004). Together with eosinophils, mast cells can also migrate *in vivo* and *in vitro* (Gruber et al. 1995) in response to VEGF, suggesting their recruitment to sites of neovascularization during physiological or pathological angiogenesis. These results indicate that a positive feed back loop can take place in allergic inflammation with Th2 mediators inducing VEGF release by eosinophils and mast cells and consequence angiogenesis, and VEGF enhancing activation of mast cells and eosinophils.

7.8 Basophils

Paul Ehrlich identified basophils in 1879 based on their unique microscopic appearance after being exposed to basic stains. Basophils are bone-marrow derived granulocytes that circulate in the peripheral blood, from where they are recruited at sites of inflammation. Their cytoplasm contains rare, small, peroxidase-positive lysosomes corresponding to azurophilic granules, and large basophilic granules, conating histamine, heparin, and leukotrienes.

Several seminal studies in the 1970s and 1980s demonstrated that basophil populations expand dramatically in response to various helminth parasites and parasite-derived antigens, suggesting that basophils might play a role in protective immunity to some parasites (Ogilvie et al. 1978).

Basophils constitutively express high affinity receptors for IgE (FcεRI), expressed on their surface. Upon interaction of this receptor-bound IgE antibodies with specific multivalent antigen, basophils undergo activation and degranulation resulting in the release of many biologically active, pro-inflammatory and/or immunoregolatory products. Basophil maturation is accompanied by an increase in methacromasia when they are stained with anionic dyes. Mature basophils are negative for naphthol AS-D chloroacetate esterase, whereas mature mast cells are positive (Parwaresch 1976).

IL-3 is an important growth factor for basophils, together with GM-CSF; IL-5 and NGF may also synergize with other growth factors to stimulate basophil maturation in vitro (Galli et al. 2001). Cytoplasmic granules of basophils contain proteoglycans, consisting of sulfated glycosaminoglycans covalently linked to a protein core. Moreover, basophils synthesize and store histamine and represent the major source of histamine present in human blood (Porter and Mitchell 1972). Basophils generate other mediators, either preformed and granule-associated (e.g. neutral proteases), or produced during activation of the cell (e.g. leukotriens, slow-reacting substances of anaphylaxis, and other metabolities of arachidonic acid and platelet-activating factor). Both mast cells and basophils exhibit amoeboid capacity, which was described as early by Maximov in 1904.

Immunologists came to recognize basophils as potential immunoregulatory cells only when it was discovered that they represent one of most potent sources of IL-4 and that they can migrate into lymph nodes to drive TH2 polarization.

In addition to their role in classic acute immediate hypersensitivity responses, e.g. anaphylaxis, mast cells and basophils can also contribute to late-phase reactions. It is widely belivied that much of the morbidity associated with chronic allergic disorders, including allergic asthma, is attributable to the actions of leukocytes recruited to the sites of late-phase reactions.

Basophils are implicated in multiple human diseases, including autoimmune disorders, inflammatory disorders, cancer, and allergies and asthma. However, the contributions of basophils to the development of human disease states remain poorly defined. Basophils are able to drive pro-inflammatory responses by recruiting effector cells such as TH2 cells, eosinophils and inflammatory macrophages to the site of inflammation.

Basophils constitutively express CCR1, CCR2, CCR3, CXCR1, CXCR3, and CXCR4 (Gibbs 2005; Min and Paul 2008). CCR3 is highly expressed on human basophils and can be activated by eotaxin (CCL11), RANTES (CCL5), MCP-3 (CCL7) and MCP-4 (CCL13) (Min et al. 2006). In contrast to human basophils, mouse basophils do not express CCR3. Upon IgE overproduction, mouse basophils release CCL22, which is a potent chemoattractant for TH2 cells and has been implicated in TH2-predominant allergic inflammation (Watanabe et al. 2008).

Basophils express mRNA for three isoforms of VEGF-A (121, 165 and 189) and two isoforms of VEGF-B (167 and 186); VEGF-A has an intracellular localization, where it co-localizes with basogranulin (Figs. 7.20, and 7.21) (de Paulis et al. 2006).

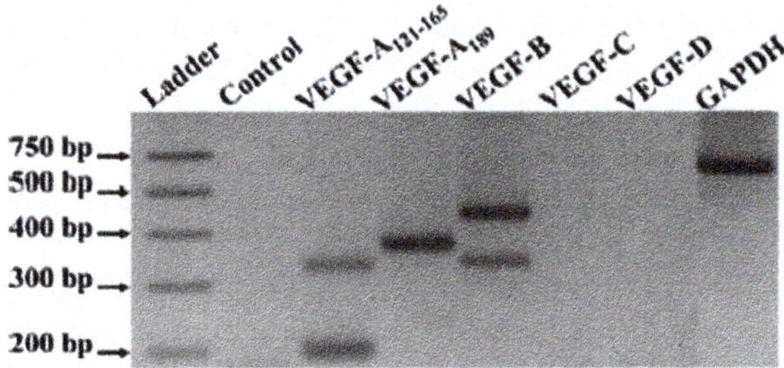

Fig. 7.20 Expression of different forms of VEGF mRNA in human basophils. Purified basophils were lysed in lysis buffer to obtain a total RNA preparation. Total RNA was reverse-transcribed and amplified by 40 PCR cycles in the presence of VEGF-specific primers and of GAPDH primers as loading control. PCR amplification of buffer represented the negative control.PCR products were analyzed by electrophoresis in 1% agarose gel containing ethidium bromide, followed by photography under UV illumination (Reproduced from de Paulis et al. 2006)

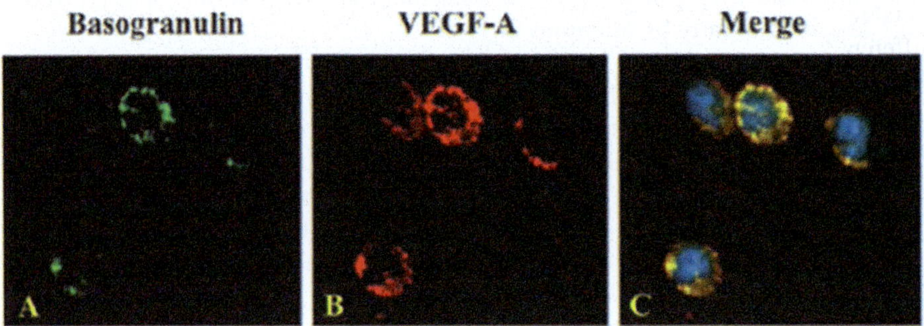

Fig. 7.21 Intracellular localization of VEGF-A in human basophils. Double immunofluorescence staining of an enriched preparation of peripheral blood basophils examined by confocal microscopy. (**a**), the intracellular localization of basogranulin by using the BB1 mAb (green); (**b**), the cells immunostained for VEGF-A (red); and (**c**), the colocalization of basogranulin and VEFG-A in human basophils (yellow) (Reproduced from de Paulis et al. 2006)

Peripheral blood and basophils infiltrating sites of chronic inflammation such as nasal polyps contain VEGF-A in their secretory granules. Supernatants of activated basophils induced an angiogenic response *in vivo* in the chick embryo CAM assay. In addition, basophils express VEGFR-2 and neuropilin-1 which acts as co-receptor for VEGFR-2 and enhances VEGFR-2-induced responses. VEGF-A also functions as basophil chemoattractant providing a novel autocrine loop for basophils self-recruitment (de Paulis et al. 2006). Human basophils express the seven-transmembrane receptor CRTH2 (chemoattractant receptor-homologous molecule expressed on TH2 cells) whose activation by PGD_2 released by mast cells induces basophil chemotaxis (Pettipher and Hansel 2008). Basophil-released histamine, in turn, may potentiate mast cell chemotaxis on the inflammatory setting by interacting with the H_4 receptor (Hofstra et al. 2003). Mast cell- and basophil-released histamine down-regulate basophil response by inhibiting the release of mediators from human basophils through engagement of the H_2 receptor (Lippert et al. 2000).

Overall, these data suggest that basophils could play a role in angiogenesis and inflammation through the expression of several forms of VEGF and their receptors. Moreover, basophils release histamine, which displays angiogenic activity in several in vitro and in vivo settings (Sorbo et al. 1994).

The precise mechanisms by which anti-IgE therapy results in reduced basophil responses and whether these effects contribute to the clinical improvement observed with anti-IgE therapy remain to be determined. Nonetheless, a better understanding of these pathways might identify biomarkers of disease severity or allow for the development of new targeted approaches for the treatment of allergic disease.

7.9 Progenitor Cells and Adult Cell Transdifferentiation

Myeloid-derived suppressor cells (MDSCs) are a heterogenous population, comprising myeloid progenitors, monocytes and neutrophils, that express low to undetectable levels of MHC-II and co-stimulatory molecules, which can further differentiate into TAMs (Fig. 7.22). MDSCs are characterized by an increased production of suppressors of T-cell functions, including reactive oxygen and nitrogen species, and by an up-regulation of the expression of arginase and inducible nitric oxide synthase (Gabrilovich and Nagaraj 2009). MDSCs can be detected in tumors as well as in the circulation of cancer patients and their number correlate with cancer stage (Almand et al. 2001).

MDSCs obtained from spleens of tumor-bearing mice promoted angiogenesis and tumor growth when co-injected with tumor cells (Yang et al. 2004). Tumors recruit MDSCs (Gabrilovich et al. 2012). Reducing the levels of MDSCs by either treatment of mice with gemcitabine or by interfering with the Kit ligand/c-Kit receptor axis impaired tumor growth and angiogenesis (Suzuki et al. 2005; Pan et al. 2007). MDSCs isolated from tumors of STAT-3-deficient mice were markedly less potent in inducing endotelial tube formation *in vitro* as compared to STAT-3 wild-

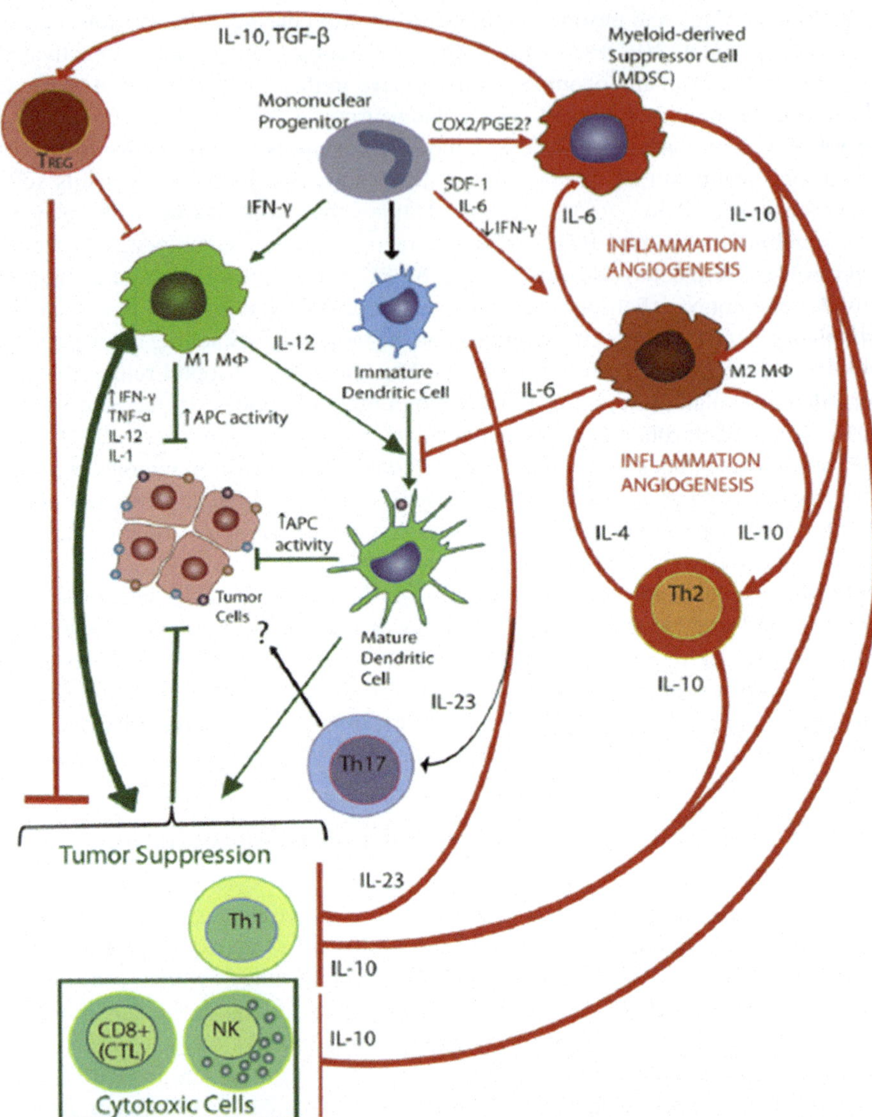

Fig. 7.22 Th2 lymphocytes, M2 macrophages and MDSCs mutually reinforce the proliferation and phenotypes of one another, as well as maintaining tumor-promoting inflammation and angiogenesis. These cells, along with T regulatory lymphocytes (TREGs) suppress the activity and proliferation of tumor-suppressing cells, including TH1, M1 and cytotoxic T cells and NK cells. TH1 and TH2 lymphocytes, as well as TREG and TH17 lymphocytes tend to self-reinforce their own activation profiles and inhibit the other (Reproduced from Burkholder et al. 2014)

type cells, concomitant with markedly reduced exepression levels of several angiogenic factors (Kujawski et al. 2008).

Upon stimulation with G-CSF, MDSCs contribute to angiogenesis by releasing Bv8 (Shojaei et al. 2007). MDSCs release MMPs that increase the bioavailability of VEGF within the tumor microenvironment (Yang et al. 2004). VEGF can promote the accumulation of MDSCs (Gabrilovich et al. 1998) and increase of MDSCs in cancer patients is correlated with the disease stage and serum VEGF levels (Almand et al. 2001). Blockade of VEGF pathway by anti-VEGF antibody in tumor-bearing mice leads to a significant reduction of MDSCs in peripheral blood as compared with untreated mice (Kusmartsev et al. 2008). A decrease in the absolute number of MDSCs in the spleen, bone marrow, and tumor in different tumor models has been observed after treatment with sunitinib (Ozao-Choy et al. 2009; Xin et al. 2009). In metastatic renal cell carcinoma patients, treatment with sunitinib decrease the percentage of MDSCs in peripheral blood (Ko et al. 2009).

Mast cells are required to enhance MDSC-mediated immune suppression and tumor escape from immune response. In a mouse model of hepatocarcinoma, infiltration and activation of mast cells lead to the mobilization of MDSCs, through CCL2 and IL-17 secretion in the tumor microenvironment (Yang et al. 2010). Moreover, mast cells induce the migration and increase the suppressive properties of splenn-derived monocytic-MDSCs through IFNγ and nitric oxide production (Danelli et al. 2004).

MDSCs seem to transdifferentiate into endothelial cell-like cells including increased expression of CD31 and VEGFR-2 and integrate into tumor vasculature (Yang et al. 2004).

7.10 Platelets

Platelets are versatile cells that play an important role in hemostasis and thrombosis and beyond. They are also actively involved in many physiological and pathological processes beyond hemostasis and thrombosis, including innate and adaptive immune responses, atherosclerosis, lymphatic vessel development, angiogenesis and tumor metastasis. Some of these processes take place at extravascular sites and are likely to be mediated by substances released by platelets.

Platelets exist in two distinct forms, resting and activated, with the resting state marked by baseline metabolic activity and the activated form resulting from agonist stimulation. Platelets possess two main secretory granules, the alpha-granules and the dense bodies, the main effectors with their highly recative and readily available contents (Table 7.7).

Platelets stimulate endothelial cell proliferation and migration, and in vivo angiogenesis, which is dependent on platelet adherence to endothelial cell through their surface adhesion molecules (Fig. 7.23) (Pipili-Synetos et al. 1998; Verheul et al. 2000a, b; Kisucka et al. 2006). Morever, platelets promote angiogenesis by

Table 7.7 Major platelet granular constituents

Alpha-granule protein
Coagulant protein (fibrinogen, factor V)
Platelet-specific proteins (platelet factor 4, β-thrombomodulin)
Mitogenic and angiogenic factors (VEGF, PDGF, TGF-β, HGF, FGF-2, EGF, CTGF)
Adhesive glycoproteins amd alpha-granule membrane-specific proteins (thrombospondin, von Willebrand factor, multimerin, P-selectin)
Dense granule constituent
Adenosine diphosphate
Calcium serotonin

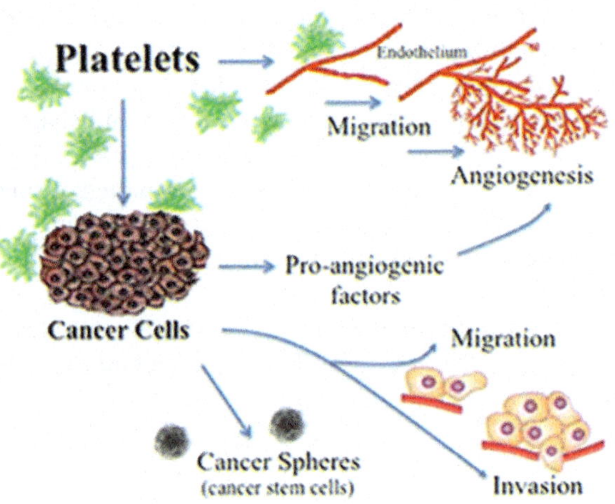

Fig. 7.23 Actions of platelets upon the processes of angiogenesis and tumor promotion. Platelets acting directly upon endothelial cells enhance the formation of tubular structures and the process of angiogenesis. Platelet acting upon the cancer cell has shown a resultant increase in the liberation of pro-angiogenic factors, an increase in cancer cell migration and invasion, and an increase in cancer sphere formation (Reproduced from Erices et al. 2017)

stimulating the mobilization of myeloid cells from the bone marrow and enhancing their homing to tumors (Feng et al. 2011).

In cultured human glioblastona multiforme cells, umbilical cord and cerebral microvascular endothelial cells, platelet-released cytokines significantly stimulate proliferation, migration and formation of capillary-like structures (Brockmann et al. 2011).

Human platelets carry in their alpha granules a set of angiogenesis stimulators, such as FGF-2, VEGF, Ang-1, HGF, PDGF, IGF-1, EGF, and thymidine phosphorylase, and inhibitors, such as endostatin, platelet factor-4 and TSP-1 (Sierko and Wojutukiewicz 2004; Italiano et al. 2007). Angiostatin was also identified in α–granules (Mc Ever 2001) and platelets membranes constitutively generate angiostatin, through a uPA-dependent mechanism (Jurasz et al. 2006). These findings may have implications for release of angiogenic molecules at the initiation of wound healing, followed by release of antiangiogenic molecules at the later stage of wound healing. These angiogenesis-regulatory molecules are packed into separate and distinc alpha-granules (Italiano et al. 2007). In fact, the treatment of human platelets with a selective proteinase activated receptor-4 (PAR-4) agonist resulted in release of endostatin-containing granules, but not VEGF-containing granules, whereas a selective PAR-1 agonist liberated VEGF, but not endostatin-containing granules (Italiano et al. 2007). These molecules are sequestered in platelets in higher concentration than in plasma. In fact, VEGF-enriched Matrigel pellets implanted subcutaneously into mice result in an elevation of VEGF levels in platelets, without any changes in its plasma levels (Klement et al. 2009). Morever, the addition of thrombin into platelet-rich plasma from healthy subjects results in much higher VEGF levels than if thrombin is added into plalelet-free plasma (Banks et al. 1998). Accumulation of platelets in some tumors and release of angiogenic molecules could further stimulate tumor growth.

ADP and thrombin receptor PAR-1 stimulation favor platelet release of pro-angiogenic regulators, whilst thromboxane A_2 (TXA_2) and PAR4 stimulation prompt selective release of anti-angiogenic regulators (Battinelli et al. 2011). The selective release of platelet pro-angiogenic regulators can be inhibited by the anticoagulants, e.g., heparins (Battinelli et al. 2014).

Platelet-derived microparticles induce angiogenesis both in vitro and in vivo and enhance vascular permeability (Brill et al. 2005; Cloutier et al. 2012). Moreover, they can transfer angiogenic factors intracellularly and induce pro-angiogenic genes in endothelial cells (Rak 2010).

Platelets isolated from cancer patients contain higher levels of pro-angiogenic factors compared with those from healthy donors (Peterson et al. 2012; Salven et al. 1999).

It has been demonstrated that accumulation of angiogenesis regulators in platelets of animals bearing malignant tumors exceeds significantly their concentration in plasma or serum, as well as their levels in platelets from non-tumor bearing mice (Klement et al. 2009). Platelets may adhere to tumor vessels, form microthrombi, and release granules that contain VEGF, PDGF together with inhibitors, such as TSP-1 and platelet factor 4.

In patients with cancer, routine tests of blood coagulation show abnormalities, including raised platelet counts, a high tumrover of platelets, and increased blood concentrations of fibrinogen breakdown products (Sun et al. 1979). Tumor endothelial cells overexpress tissue factor (TF) and positive correlations between TF expression and vascular density or TF and VEGF-A expression have been observed in different tumors (Sabrkhany et al. 2011).

Notodihardjo et al. (2015) demonstrated that gelatin hydrogel impregnated with platelet-rich plasma releasate promotes angiogenesis and wound healing in a murine model. Ang-1 is highly expressed in platelet-rich plasma (Mammoto et al. 2013). Moreover, inhibition of Ang-1 Tie-2 signalling suppress the angiogenic induction by a platelet-rich fibrin matrix in vivo.

7.11   Fibroblasts

In the specific context of solid tumors, fibroblasts are referred as cancer associated fibroblasts (CAFs) or tumor associated fibroblasts (TAFs) and exhibit some similarities with myofibroblasts, originally characterized in wound healing and fibrosis (Gabbiani et al. 1971; Madar et al. 2013). In breast, prostate, and pancreatic carcinomas, CAFs parallel higher malignancy grade, tumor progression, and poor prognosis (Kalluru and Zeisberg 2006; Franco et al. 2010; Orimoa and Weinberg 2006; Shimoda et al. 2010. In mouse xenografts, CAFs inoculated with carcinoma cells promote tumor survival, proliferation and invasive behaviour (Erez et al. 2010; Orimo et al. 2005).

The definition of CAFs encompasses a few important features: (i) these fibroblasts are in close contact with cancer cells, (ii) CAFs display peculiar immunophenotypic and functional features that sharply differentiate them from normal, resting fibroblasts located in non-neoplastic environments, and (iii) the properties acquired by CAFs upon interaction with cancer cells render them supportive of tumor growth and progression through different mechanisms including extracellular matrix remodelling, cell proliferation, angiogenesis and epithelial mesenchymal transition (EMT) (Cirri and Chiarugi 2012).

CAF activation is commonly accompanied by the acquisition or upregulation of specific markers which can be classified in four groups: (i) the fibroblast activation markers, which include fibroblast specific protein (FSP) and fibroblast activation protein (FAP); (ii) the aggressiveness markers thrombospondin-1 (TSP-1), tenascin-C and stromelysin; (iii) the pro-angiogenic markers (desmin-1, FGF-2, alpha smooth-muscle-actin (α-SMA) and VEGF); and (iv) the growth factors that support tumor growth and inflammation (EGF, HGF, IL-6, FGF-2 (Cirri and Chiarugi 2012; Räsänen and Vaheri 2010). Moreover, CAFs express MMP1, MMP-3, produce collagens, and release cytokines and pro-angiogenic growth factors (Kopp et al. 2005), including VEGF, HGF, FGF-2, Ang-1, IL-6, IL-8, MCP-1, identified within in vitro secretome of adult tissue-derived MSCs (Chen et al. 2008). CAFs are a major source of VEGF in transgenic mice (Fukumura et al. 1998), and CAF-derived VEGF enhances the expression and activation of integrins (Byzova et al. 2000). CAF-derived PDGF sustains angiogenesis by further stimulating CAFs to secrete pro-angiogenic growth factors, including FGF-2 and osteopontin (Pietras et al. 2008; Anderberg et al. 2009).

CAFs release angiogenic factors through proteolysis of the extracellular matrix. In this respect, CAFs localized in invasive human breast carcinomas promote tumor growth and angiogenesis through elevated Stromal-Derived-factor-1 (SDF-1)/CXCL12 secretion (Orimo et al. 2005).

Co-implantation of CAFs and cancer cells enhances angiogenesis, decreases cancer cell dormancy and accelerates tumor growth in mice (Tuxhorn et al. 2002; Orimo et al. 2005).

The heterogeneity in marker expression led to hypothesize that CAFs could have multiple origins, depending on the tumor histotype and the area of the neoplastic lesion (De Wever et al. 2014). Indeed, it is becoming evident that CAFs originate from local or distant reservoirs through different types of trans differentiation processes.

The primary source of CAFs is represented by resident fibroblast or pericytes which trans differentiate through a mesenchymal-mesenchymal transition (MMT) driven by specific cancer-derived factors such as TGF-β, PDGF, FGF-2, and SDF-1 (Fig. 7.24) (Cirri and Chiarugi 2011; Kojima et al. 2010). In addition, CAFs may originate from local epithelial normal and transformed cells that transdifferentiate through an EMT into activated fibroblasts (Radisky et al. 2007; Weber et al. 2003). These findings were also supported by the observation that stromal cells of breast tumors shared genetic lesions in common with tumor epithelium (Kurose et al., 2002; Moinfar et al., 2000). EMT that gives origin to CAFs often occurs in epithelial cells that acquire mutations following oxidative stress (Radisky et al. 2005). In

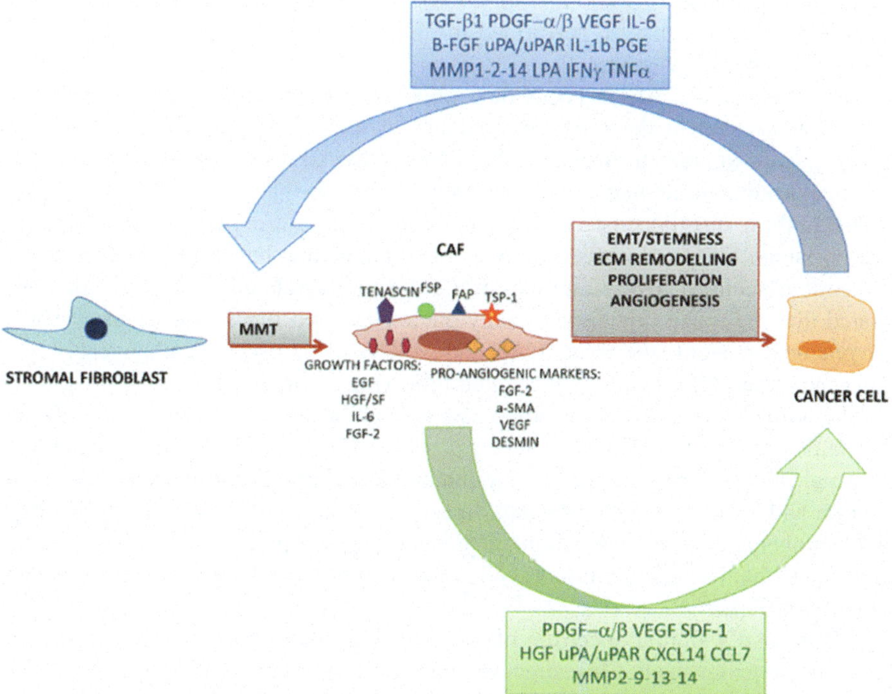

Fig. 7.24 Interaction between CAFs and cancer cells. Cancer-derived factors induce a Mesenchymal Mesenchymal Transition (MMT) through which resident normal fibroblast are activated and acquire the expression of various markers such as tenascin, fibroblast specific protein (FSP), fibroblast activation protein (FAP), thrombospondin-1 (TSP-1) and pro-angiogenic molecules. In turn, CAFs secrete various growth factors which sustain tumor progression by promoting Epithelial Mesenchymal Transition (EMT), stemness, extracellular matrix remodeling, proliferation and angiogenesis (Reproduced from Raffaghello et al. 2014)

this regard, a study reported that MMP-3 promotes EMT by inducing the expression of an alternatively spliced form of Rac1, which causes an increase in cellular reactive oxygen species (ROS) and consequently oxidative damage to DNA and genomic instability (Radisky et al. 2005). On the contrary, other studies demonstrated that somatic mutations can occur exclusively in cancer cells and that CAF mutations are a very rare event (Qiu et al. 2008). Similarly to EMT, CAFs may also derive from local endothelial cells through an EndMT mainly driven by tumor-derived TGF-β. During this process, endothelial cells loose the expression of CD31 and acquire that of mesenchymal cells like α-SMA and FSP-1 (Zeisberg et al. 2007).

Bone marrow and adipose tissue represent two distant sites that significantly contribute to CAF generation (De Wever et al. 2014). In particular, cancer-derived soluble factors recruit MSCs to tumor sites, where the latter cells acquire the expression of CAF-specific markers such as α-SMA, FAP, tenascin-C and TSP-1 (Kidd et al. 2012; Spaeth et al. 2009). More importantly, in tumor microenvironment MSCs exhibit typical functional properties of CAFs, including high expression of SDF-1 and the ability to promote tumor cell growth both *in vitro* and in *in vivo* coimplantation models (Mishra et al. 2008). It is of note that most of the studied regarding CAF origin were performed in mouse tumors. In contrast, information from human tumors is scarse.

The definition of CAFs has become popular and widely used to indicate activated fibroblasts present in the microenvironment of most solid tumors, whereas it is rarely utilized to indicate stromal cells of mesenchymal origin found in the specific microenvironments of hematopoietic malignancies, i.e. bone marrow and lymph nodes. In these disorders, such stromal cells are often referred to as MSCs or, more appropriately, MSCs. However the few comparisons that have been done between leukemia-associated MSCs and classical solid tumor-related CAFs have demonstrated that these cell types share many phenotypic and functional features. Thus, for practical reasons, the terms CAF and MSC will be used interchangeably, the latter indicating MSCs usually generated following *in vitro* culture.

The primary functions of fibroblasts are the synthesis and deposition of collagen that builds up the scaffold of connective tissues (Gabbiani et al. 1971; Cirri and Chiarugi, 2012). CAFs acquire a new functional polarization translating into production and release of proteases that digest the extracellular matrix (e.g. MMPs), pro-angiogenic factors that stimulate microvessel formation and pro-metastatic molecules that accelerate tumor cell dissemination to distant sites (Cirri and Chiarugi 2012).

MSCs have a similar spectrum of activities but, in contrast to fibroblasts, they have been extensively investigated for their immunoregulatory properties (Barcellos-de Souza et al. 2013; Uccelli et al. 2008). Nonetheless, the few studies that have addressed the immumodulatory activities of classic fibroblasts of mesodermal origin have shown that the latter behave as MSCs. Since cancer-driven immunosuppression is one of the key step to create a pro-tumoral microenvironment, we will summarize the state of the art of the immunosuppressive activities of MSCs assuming that fibroblasts in general and especially CAFs share these feature with MSCs.

7.11.1 Therapeutic Strategies

Given their relevant role in driving tumor progression, CAFs have been emerged as therapeutic targets by various strategies reported. The interplay between CAFs and cancer cells is characterized by a feed-forward loop in which various growth factors/cytokines and their receptors play an important role in promoting tumor growth and progression. If on one side tumor cells secrete a plethora of factors such as TGF-β1, PDGF, VEGF, IL-6, FGF-2, IFN-γ, TNF, MMPs involved in fibroblast activation, on the other side, CAFs produce the same molecules affecting tumor aggressiveness. In this context, several strategies have been designed to target the growth factors and their receptors by the use of antagonists or specific antibodies that, in some cases, may act simultaneously on tumor cells and CAFs. For example, the recent FDA approved pazopanib (Votrient), a multi target receptor tyrosine kinase inhibitor (TKI) against PDGFR β, VEGFR-1, −2, −3 and c-kit (Escudier et al. 2014), as well as MET/HGF inhibitors (monoclonal antibodies against HGF and selective MET tyrosine kinase inhibitors) (Rosen et al. 2010) and the humanized monoclonal antibody (mAb) against VEGF-A Bevacizumab (Avastin) (Ebos and Kerbel 2011) have been validated to target the same molecules expressed by tumor cells and CAFs. Particular interest has been focused on specific blockers of PDGF and HGF receptor signalling in CAFs, that demonstrated to inhibit tumor growth and progression in preclinical tumor models (Kim et al. 2006; Pietras et al. 2008; Wen et al. 2004).

Another approach has been designed to target the urokinase plasminogen activation (uPA) uPA/uPA receptor (R) system that represents one of the key systems driving tumor invasion and metastases (Smith and Marshall 2010). uPAR is frequently overexpressed in cancer cells and tumor-associated stromal cells such as CAFs, is associated to poor prognosis and in some cases is predictive of invasion and metastasis (Bene et al. 2004; Jacobsen and Ploug 2008). Thus, new uPAR-targeted therapies might be effective against both tumor cells and cells of the tumor microenvironment. Several therapeutic approaches aimed at inhibiting the uPA/uPAR, such as selective inhibitors of uPA activity, antagonist peptides, mAb able to prevent uPA binding to uPAR and gene therapy techniques silencing uPA/uPAR expression functions, have been shown to possess anti-tumor effects in xenograft models (Ulisse et al. 2009). However, all these strategies need definitive confirmation in humans as only few uPA inhibitors entered clinical trial.

Another interesting approach concerns the use of inhibitors of COX-2, an inflammatory molecule overexpressed in both CAFs and tumor cells upon their reciprocal interaction (Greenhough et al. 2009; Sato et al. 2004). COX-2 promotes tumor progression by inducing EMT and stimulating VEGF-mediated angiogenesis and MMP-14-driven invasion (Cattaruzza et al. 2009; Giannoni et al. 2010). In this respect, preclinical and clinical trials demonstrated that COX-2 inhibitors such as Celecoxib (Celebrex) represent a promising strategy in the prevention and treatment of solid tumors (Ghosh et al. 2010).

Given the relevant role of MMPs in promoting tumor invasiveness and metastasis, great efforts have been made in order to develop specific MMP inhibitors (Chen et al. 2008). The most extensively studied classes of MMP inhibitors include Batimastat, Marismastat, Prinomastat and Tanomastat that are currently undergoing clinical trial in several malignant and malignant diseases (Chaudhary et al. 2010). However, their efficacy and action have not been confirmed and more data are required.

FAP, a member of the serine protease family, selectively expressed on CAFs and cancer cells, exerts a proteolytic activity that supports tumor growth and proliferation (Liu et al. 2012). Thus, FAP has been considered as an emerging novel therapeutic target in cancer. A humanized anti-FAP antibody (mAb F19; sibrotuzumab) is well tolerated (Scott et al. 2003) but it showed no beneficial effect in a phase II trial for metastatic colorectal cancer (Hofheinz et al. 2003). It was reported that a monoclonal anti-FAP antibody conjugated to maytansinoid induced a long-lasting inhibition of tumor growth and complete regression in different experimental tumor models, without signs of toxicity (Ostermann et al. 2008). However, further studies are required to determine the clinical application.

An interesting approach to target CAFs focuses on the development of specific antibodies against integrins, that have been found to be expressed by tumor cells and CAFs and to be involved in cancer progression (Desgrosellier and Cheresh 2010). In particular, a recent study demonstrated that integrin $\alpha v \beta 6$ leads to CAFs proliferation, and consequently increases gastric cancer metastasis (Zhang et al. 2013). Furthermore, a human therapeutic antibody 264RAD, which binds to $\alpha v \beta 6$ and inhibits its function, has been shown to delay tumor growth by preventing TGF-β-mediated activation of CAFs, and by reducing the expression of fibronectin and a-SMA on stromal fibroblasts (Eberlein et al. 2013). Therefore, disruption of the expression of integrin $\alpha v \beta 6$ may be a new target for future cancer therapy.

Finally, curcumine has been demonstrated as a molecule able to target the dynamic mutual interaction between CAFs and head and neck tumor cells (Dudas et al. 2013). Specifically, curcumin reduced the release of EMT-mediators by CAFs with consequent reduction of cancer invasion. These data confirmed the potential of curcumin in clinical application and underline the need of improved formulation for *in vivo* delivery.

Chapter 8
Conclusions

Experimental and clinical data indicate that plasticity is a common property of most leukocyte subtypes and thus can be targeted therapeutically. Monocyte/macrophage phenotype switching from a pro- to anti-angiogenic secretory profile is crucial for vessel remodeling and therapeutic immune effects (De Palma and Lewis 2013). Tumor-targeted IFNα delivery by TEMs reduces angiogenesis in murine breast and brain cancer models (De Palma et al. 2008). Anti-VEGF treatment in murine melanoma synergizes with adoptive T cell transfer by increasing leukocyte access into tumors and enhance the effectiveness of adoptive immunotherapy (Shrimali et al. 2010). Low dose VEGFR-2 blockade increases the efficacy of anti-tumor vaccination in breast cancer models by generating M1 macrophage and facilitating effector T cell infiltration (Huang et al. 2012).

Development of therapies to prevent the adverse effects of cancer-causing pathogens, such as vaccines against hepatitis B viruses and human papilloma virus, contribute to decreasing morbidity from hepatocellular and cervical carcinoma, respectively (Porta et al. 2011). Eradication of chronic *Helycobacter Pylori* infection with antimicrobials is likely to reduce the incidence of gastric cancer (Porta et al. 2011).

A number of anti-oxidant anti-inflammatory drugs have anti-angiogenic potential by acting on inflammation-mediated angiogenesis (Albini et al. 2005). Anti inflammatory drugs, including aspirin, non steroidal anti inflammatory drugs (NSAIDs), cyclooxygenase −2 (COX-2) inhibitors (e.g. celecoxib), and glucocorticoids (e.g. dexamethasone) have been demonstrated to reduce tumor incidence or progression and reduce mortality (Clevers 2004; Porta et al. 2011). The NSAIDs exert their anti-inflammatory and anti-tumor effects mainly by inhibiting the action of COX-2 leading to a reduced production of prostaglandins, promoting an infiltration of inflammatory cells, creating a favourable microenvironment for tumor progression (Zha et al. 2004).

COX-2 inhibitors inhibit angiogenesis in tumor growth ulcers, and granulation tissue (Monnier et al. 2005). Rapamycin, an inhibitor of mTOR (mammalian target of rapamycin) is a natural macrolide antibiotic used as immunosuppressive agent

© Springer International Publishing AG 2017

D. Ribatti, *Inflammation and Angiogenesis*, https://doi.org/10.1007/978-3-319-68448-2_8

after organ transplantation (Motzer et al. 2008). Rapamycin inhibits primary and metastatic tumor growth by anti angiogenesis (Guba et al. 2002; Marimpietri et al. 2005, 2007; Xue et al. 2009). A bisphosphonate compound, zoledronic acid, inhibits in vitro endothelial cell proliferation and migration, and capillarogenesis of bone marrow endothelial cells of patients with multiple myeloma, and angiogenesis in vivo in the chorioallantoic membrane assay (Scavelli et al. 2007).

Bisphosphonate-mediated inhibition of MMP-9 decreased angiogenesis in human tumor xenografts (Huang et al. 2009) and in a mouse model of human papilloma virus 16 (HPV16)-driven cervical cancer (Giraudo et al. 2004).

Some analysts have predicted that within 10 years, immunotherapy will constitute 60% of all cancer treatments (Ledford 2014). A novel group of immunomodulatory antibodies has been introduced in the clinical use, which can break tumor specific immune tolerance and induce regression of tumors. These antibodies block growth signals of tumor cells, or induce apoptosis. Since the introduction of rituximab (Cheson and Leonard 2008), 13 further tumor-directed antibodies have been approved.

Anti-TNF therapy, including TNF monoclonal blocking antibodies (infliximab, adalimumab, certolizumab, pegol and golimumab), or soluble TNF receptor fusion proteins (etanercept) results in vessel stabilization and normalization (Izquierdo et al. 2009). Il-17 contributes to both angiogenesis through VEGF expression and other pathological processes in chronic inflammatory disorders. IL-17 induced tumors to release CSF-3, which promotes VEGF-A-independent tumor vascularization (Chung et al. 2013). IL-17 blocking therapies (secukinumab and ixekizumab) exert anti-angiogenic activities (Van Den Berg and MCInnes 2013; Baeten et al. 2015). Moreover, blocking IL-17 render tumors more susceptible to anti-angiogenic therapies (Chung et al. 2013). Esalazine, a drug often used in ulcerative colitis, inhibits NF, downregulates angiostatiand endostatin, lowers MMP-2 and MMP-9 levels (Deng et al. 2009).

Three of the most significant therapeutic approaches are represented by sipuleucel-T, an immunotherapeutic vaccine for prostate cancer (Gulley et al. 2015); ipilimumab, a check point inhibitor of CTLA-4 (Hodi et al. 2010), and anti-programmed death receptor-1 (PD-1) and its ligand PDL-1 antibodies (anti-PD-1/PD-L-1) (He et al. 2004; Blank et al. 2004; Philips and Atkins 2015) for the treatment of metastatic melanoma.

Cancer immunotherapies are classified as active and passive treatments. Active treatments include vaccines designed to induce tumor cell recognition. Passive treatments, on the other hand, imply direct administration of antibodies and T cells, to the patient. In this context, immune checkpoint inhibitors and adoptive T cell therapy are among the most innovative approaches (Sharma and Allison 2015). At the clinical level, it is not yet clarified why certain patients respond to specific types of immunotherapies, while others do not. The development of future treatments depends on finding effective immune-based biomarkers that can help to predict responses to treatment. Combination of immunosuppressant with anti-angiogenic drugs may be beneficial in patients not responding to conventional treatments.

References

Abdel-Majid RM, Marshall JS (2004) Prostaglandin E2 induces degranulation-independent production of vascular endothelial growth factor by human mast cells. J Immunol 172:1227–1236

Afzal A, Shaw LC, Ljubimov AV et al (2007) Retinal and choroidal microangiopathies: therapeutic opportunities. Microvasc Res 74:131–144

Aharjnejad S, Abraham D, Paulus P et al (2002) Colonystimulating factor-1 antisense treatment suppresses growth of human tumor xenografts in mice. Cancer Res 62:5317–5324

Aharjnejad S, Paulus P, Sioud M et al (2004) Colony-stimulating factor-1 blockade by antisense oligonucleotide and small interfering RNAs suppresses growth of human mammary tumor xenograft in mice. Cancer Res 64:5387–5394

Ai S, Cheng XW, Inoue A et al (2007) Angiogenic activity of bFGF and VEGF suppressed by proteolytic cleavage by neutrophil elastase. Biochem Biophys Res Commun 364:395–401

Albini A, Tosetti F, Benelli E et al (2005) Tumor inflammatory angiogenesis and its chemoprevention. Cancer Res 65:10637–10641

Almand B, Clark JI, Nikitina E et al (2001) Increased production of immature myeloid cells in cancer patients: a mechanism of immunosuppression in cancer. J Immunol 166:678–689

Ancelin M, Chollet-Martin S, Hervé MA et al (2004) Vascular endothelial growth factor VEGF189 induces human neutrophil chemotaxis in extravascular tissue via an autocrine amplification mechanism. Lab Investig 84:502–512

Anderberg C, Li H, Fredriksson L et al (2009) paracrine signaling by platelet-derived growth factor CC promotes tumor growth by recruitment of cancer-associated fibroblasts. Cancer Res 69:368–378

Andreu P, Johansson M, Affara NI et al (2010) FcRγ Activation Regulates Inflammation-Associated Squamous Carcinogenesis. Cancer Cell 17:121–134

Aoki M, Pawankar R, Niimi Y et al (2003) Mast cells in basal cell carcinoma express VEGF, IL-8 and RANTES. Int Arch Allergy Immunol 130:216–223

Ardi VC, Kupriyanova TA, Deryugina EI et al (2007) Human neutrophils uniquely release TIMP-free MMP-9 to provide a potent catalytic stimulator of angiogenesis. Proc Natl Acad Sci U S A 104:20262–20267

Aroni K, Tsagroni E, Kavantzas N et al (2007) A study of the pathogenesis of Rosacea: how angiogenesis and mast cells may participate in a complex multifactorial process. Arch Dermatol Res 300:125–131

Asai K, Kanazawa H, Otani K et al (2002) Imbalance between vascular endothelial growth factor and endostatin levels in induced sputum from asthmatic subjects. J Allergy Clin Immunol 110:571–575

© Springer International Publishing AG 2017

D. Ribatti, *Inflammation and Angiogenesis*, https://doi.org/10.1007/978-3-319-68448-2

Assoian RK, Fleurdelys BE, Stevenson HC et al (1987) Expression and secretion of type beta transforming growth factor by activated human macrophages. Proc Natl Acad Sci U S A 84:6020–6024

Auerbach R (1988) Patterns of tumor metastasis: organ selectivity in the spread of cancer cells. Lab Investig 58:361–364

Auerbach R, Alby L, Morrissey LW et al (1985) Expression of organ-specific antigens on capillary endothelial cells. Microvasc Res 29:401–411

Auerbach R, Lu WC, Pardon E et al (1987) Specificity of adhesion between murine tumor cells and capillary endothelium: an in vitro correlate of preferential metastasis in vivo. Cancer Res 47:1492–1496

Augustin HG, Young Koh G, Thurston G et al (2009) Control of vascular morphogenesis and homeostasis through the angiopoietin-Tie system. Nat Rev Mol Cell Biol 10:165–177

Aurora AB, Baluk P, Zhang D et al (2005) Immune complex-dependent remodeling of the airway vasculature in response to a chronic bacterial infection. J Immunol 175:6319–6326

Avraham-Davidi I, Yona S, Grunewald M et al (2013) On-site education of VEGF-recruited monocytes improves their performance as angiogenic and arteriogenic accessory cells. J Exp Med 210:2611–2625

Azenshtein E, Luboshits G, Shina S et al (2002) The CC chemokine RANTES in breast carcinoma progression: regulation of expression and potential mechanisms of promalignant activity. Cancer Res 62:1093–1102

Baer C, Squadrito ML, Laoui D et al (2016) Suppression of microRNA activity amplifies IFN-gamma-induced macrophage activation and promotes anti-tumor immunity. Nat Cell Biol 18:790–802

Baeten D, Sieper J, Barun J et al (2015) Secukinumab, an interleukin-17 inhibitor, in ankyylosing spondylitis. N Engl J Med 373:2534–2548

Baird A, Mormède P, Böhlen P (1985) Immunoreactive fibroblast growth factor in cells of peritoneal exudate suggests its identity with macrophage-derived growth factor. Biochem Biophys Res Commun 126:358–364

Balkwill FR (1992) Tumour necrosis factor and cancer. Prog Growth Factor Res 4:121–137

Balkwill F (2002) Tumor necrosis factor or tumor promoting factor? Cytokine Growth Factor Rev 13:135–141

Balkwill F, Mantovani A (2001) Inflammation and cancer: back to Virchow? Lancet 357:539–545

Balkwill F, Charles KA, Mantovani A (2005) Smoldering and polarized inflammation in the initiation and promotion of malignant disease. Cancer Cell 7:211–217

Banchereau J, Steinman RM (1998) Dendritic cells and the control of immunity. Nature 392:245–252

Banchereau J, Briere F, Caux C et al (2000) Immunobiology of dendritic cells. Annu Rev Immunol 18:767–811

Banks RE, Forbes MA, Kinsey SE et al (1998) Release of the angiogenic cytokine vascular endothelial growth factor (VEGF) from platelets: significance for VEGF measurements and cancer biology. Br J Cancer 77:956–964

Barcellos-de-Souza P, Gori V, Bambi F et al (2013) Tumor microenvironment: bone marrow-msenchymal stem cells as key players. Biochim Biophys Acta 1863:321–335

Barrera P, Blom A, Van Lent PLEM et al (2000) Synovial macrophage depletion with clodronate-containing liposomes in rheumatoid arthritis. Arthritis Rheum 43:1951–1959

Bartlett MR, Underwood PA, Parish CR (1995) Comparative analysis of the ability of leucocytes, endothelial cells and platelets to degrade the subendothelial basement membrane: Evidence for cytokine dependence and detection of a novel sulfatase. Immunol Cell Biol 73:113–124

Battinelli EM, Markens BA, Italiano JE Jr (2011) Release of angiogenesis regulatory proteins from platelet alpha granules: modulation of physiologic and pathologic angiogenesis. Blood 118:1359–1369

Battinelli EM, Markens BA, Kulenthirarajan RA et al (2014) Anticoagulation inhibits tumor cell-mediated release of platelet angiogenic proteins and diminishes platelet angiogenic response. Blood 123:101–112

Baumann M et al (2008) Exploring the role of cancer stem cells in radioresistance. Nat Rev Cancer 8:545–554

Bazzoni F, Cassatella MA, Rossi F et al (1991) Phagocytosing neutrophils produce and release high amounts of the neutrophil-activating peptide 1/interleukin 8. J Exp Med 173:771–774

Belardelli F, Ferrantini M (2002) Cytokines as a link between innate and adaptive antitumor immunity. Trends Immunol 23:201–208

Bene MC, Castoldi G, Knapp W et al (2004) CD87 (urokinase-type plasminogen activator receptor), function and pathology in hematological disorders: a review. Leukemia 18:394–400

Benelli R, Morini M, Carrozzino F et al (2002) Neutrophils as a key cellular target for angiostatin: implications for regulation of angiogenesis and inflammation. FASEB J 16:267–269

Benitez-Bribiesca L, Wong A, Utrera D et al (2001) The role of mast cell tryptase in neoangiogenesis of premalignant and malignant lesions of the uterine cervix. J Histochem Cytochem 49:1061–1062

Berse B, Brown LF, Van de Water L et al (1992) Vascular permeability factor (vascular endothelial growth factor) gene is expressed differentially in normal tissues, macrophages, and tumors. Mol Biol Cell 3:211–220

Bezuidenhout L, Bracher M, Davison G et al (2007) Ang-2 and PDGF-BB cooperatively stimulate human peripheral blood monocyte fibrinolysis. J Leukoc Biol 81:1496–1503

Bingle L, Brown NJ, Lewis CE (2002) The role of tumour-associated macrophages in tumour progression: implications for new anticancer therapies. J Pathol 196:254–265

Bingle L, Lewis CE, Corke K et al (2005) Macrophages promote angiogenesis in human breast tumour spheroids in vivo. Br J Cancer 94:101–107

Biswas SK, Mantovani A (2010) Macrophage plasticity and interaction with lymphocyte substets: cancer as a paradigm. Nat Immunol 11:889–896

Blair RJ, Meng H, Marchese MJ et al (1997) Human mast cells stimulate vascular tube formation. Tryptase is a novel, potent angiogenic factor. J Clin Invest 99:2691–2700

Blank C, Brown I, Peterson AC et al (2004) PD-L1/B7H-1 inhibits the effector phase of tumor rejection by T cell receptor (TCR) transgenic CD8+ T cells. Cancer Res 64:1140–1145

Blotnick S, Peoples GE, Freeman MR et al (1994) T lymphocytes synthesize and export heparin-binding epidermal growth factor-like growth factor and basic fibroblast growth factor, mitogens for vascular cells and fibroblasts: differential production and release by CD4+ and CD8+ T cells. Proc Natl Acad Sci U S A 91:2890–2894

Bochner BS, Charlesworth EN, Lichtenstein LM et al (1990) Interleukin-1 is released at sites of human cutaneous allergic reactions. J Allergy Clin Immunol 86:830–839

Boesiger J, Tsai M, Maurer M et al (1998) Mast cells can secrete vascular permeability factor/vascular endothelial cell growth factor and exhibit enhanced release after immunoglobulin E–dependent upregulation of Fcε receptor I expression. J Exp Med 188:1135–1145

Dolitho P, Street SEA, Westwood JA et al (2009) Perforin-mediated suppression of B-cell lymphoma. Proc Natl Acad Sci U S A 106:2723–2728

Boon T, van der Bruggen P (1996) Human tumor antigens recognized by T lymphocytes. J Exp Med 183:725–729

Bosco MC, Puppo M, Blengio F et al (2008) Monocytes and dendritic cells in an hypoxic environment: spotlights in chemotaxis and migration. Immunobiology 213:733–749

Bottazzi B, Polentarutti N, Acero R et al (1983) Regulation of the macrophage content of neoplasms by chemoattractants. Science 220:210–212

Bourbie-Vaudaine S, Blanchard N, Hivroz C et al (2006) Dendritic cells can turn CD4+ T lymphocytes into vascular endothelial growth factor-carrying cells by intercellular neuropilin-1 transfer. J Immunol 177:1460–1469

Bowrey PF, King J, Magarey C et al (2000) Histamine, mast cells and tumour cell proliferation in breast cancer: does preoperative cimetidine administration have an effect? Br J Cancer 82:167–170

Bradding P, Feather IH, Wilson S et al (1993) Immunolocalization of cytokines in the nasal mucosa of normal and perennial rhinitic subjects. The mast cell as a source of IL-4, IL-5, and IL-6 in human allergic mucosal inflammation. J Immunol 151:3853–3865

Brill A, Dashevsky O, Rivo J et al (2005) Platelet-derived microparticles induce angiogenesis and stimulate post-ischaemic revascularization. Cardiovasc Res 67:30–38

Brockmann MA, Bender B, Plaxina E et al (2011) Differential effects of tumor-platelet interaction in vitro and in vivo in glioblastoma. J Neuro-Oncol 105:45–56

Bruno A, Focaccetti C, Pagani A et al (2013) The pro-angiogenic phenotype of natural killer cells in patients with non small cell lung cancer. Neoplasia 15:133–142

Bruno A, Ferlazzo G, Albini A et al (2014) A think tank of TINK/TANKs: tumor-infiltrating / tumor-associated natural killer cells in tumor progression and angiogenesis. J Natl Cancer Inst 106:dju200

Burke B, Giannoudis A, Corke KP et al (2003) Hypoxia-induced gene expression in human macrophages: implications for ischemic tissues and hypoxia-regulated gene therapy. Am J Pathol 163:1233–1243

Burkholder B, Huang RY, Burgess R et al (2014) Tumor-induced perturbations of cytokines andimmune cell networks. Biochimica et Biophysica Acta 1845:182–201

Burnet FM (1957) Cancer; a biological approach. I. The processes of control. Br Med J 1:779–782

Burnet FM (1970) Immunological surveillance. Pergamon Press, Oxford

Byzova TV, Goldman CK, Pampori N et al (2000) A mechanism for modulation of cellular responses to VEGF: activation of the integrins. Mol Cell 6:851–861

Cacalano G, Lee J, Kikly K et al (1994) Neutrophil and B cell expansion in mice that lack the murine IL-8 receptor homolog. Science 265:682–684

Candido J, Hagemann T (2013) Cancer-related inflammmation. J Clin Immunol 33(suppl 1):79–84

Capoccia BJ, Gregory AD, Link DC (2008) Recruitment of the inflammatory subset of monocytes to sites of ischemia induces angiogenesis in a monocyte chemoattractant protein-1-dependent fashion. J Leukoc Biol 84:760–768

Carmeliet P, Tessier-Lavigne M (2005) Common mechanisms of nerve and blood vessel wiring. Nature 436:193–200

Cattaruzza L, Gloghini A, Olivo K et al (2009) Functional coexpression of Interleukin (IL)-7 and its receptor (IL-7R) on Hodgkin and Reed-Sternberg cells: involvement of IL-7 in tumor cell growth and microenvironmental interactions of Hodglin's lymphoma. Int J Cancer 125:1092–1101

Cavallo F, Quaglino E, Cifaldi L et al (2001) Interleukin 12-activated lymphocytes influence tumor genetic programs. Cancer Res 61:3518–3523

Chambers AF, Groom AC, Mac Donald IC (2002) Dissemination and growth of cancer cells in metastatic sites. Nat Rev Cancer 2:563–572

Chambers SE, O'Neill CL, O'Dohy TM et al (2013) The role of immune-related myeloid cells in angiogenesis. Immunobiology 218:1370–1375

Chapman JR, Webster AC, Wong W (2013) Cancer in the transplant recipient. Cold Spring Harb Perspect Med 3:a015677

Chaudhary AK, Singh M, Bharti AC et al (2010) Genetic polymorphism of matrix metalloproteinases and their inhibitors in potentially malignant and malignant lesions of the head and neck. J Biomed Sci 17:10–20

Chavakis T, Cines DB, Rhee JS et al (2004) Regulation of neovascularization by human neutrophil peptides (alpha-defensins): a link between inflammation and angiogenesis. FASEB J 18:1306–1308

Chen L, Tredget EE, Wu PY et al (2008) Paracrine factors of mesenchymal stem cells recruit macrophages and endothelial lineage cells and enhance wound healing. PLoS One 3, e1886

Cheng SS, Kunkel SL (2003) The evolving role of neutrophils in chemokine networks. Chem Immunol Allergy 83:81–94

Cheson BD, Leonard JP (2008) Monoclonal antibody therapy for B-cell non Hodgkin's lymphoma. N Engl J Med 359:613–626

Chetta A, Zanini A, Olivieri D (2007) Therapeutic approach to vascular remodelling in asthma. Pulm Pharmacol Ther 20:1–8

Chung AS, Wu X, Zhuang G et al (2013) An interleukin-17-mediated paracrine network promotes tumor resistance to anti-angiogenic therapy. Nat Med 19:1114–1123

Cirri P, Chiarugi P (2011) Cancer associated fibroblasts: the dark side of the coin. Am J Cancer Res 1:482–497

Cirri P, Chiarugi P (2012) Cancer-associated fibroblasts and tumour cells: a diabolic liaison driving cancer progression. Cancer Metastasis Rev 31:195–208

Clauss M, Gerlach M, Gerlach H et al (1990) Vascular permeability factor: a tumor-derived polypeptide that induces endothelial cell and monocyte procoagulant activity, and promotes monocyte migration. J Exp Med 172:1535–1545

Clemente CG, Mihm MC Jr, Bufalino R (1996) Prognostic value of tumor infiltrating lymphocytes in the vertical growth phase of primary cutaneous melanoma. Cancer 77:1303–1310

Clementi R, Locatelli F, Dupré L et al (2005) A proportion of patients with lymphoma may harbor mutations of the perforin gene. Blood 105:4424–4428

Clevers H (2004) At the crossroads of inflammation and cancer. Cell 118:671–674

Cloutier N, Pare A, Farndale RW et al (2012) Platelets can enhance vascular permeability. Blood 120:1334–1343

Coffelt SB, Wellenstein MD, de Visser KE (2016) Neutrophils in cancer: neutral no more. Nat Rev Cancer 16:431–446

Colombo MP, Trinchieri G (2002) Interleukin-12 in anti-tumor immunity and immunotherapy. Cytokine Growth Factor Res 13:155–168

Conley SJ, Gheordunescu E, Kakarala P et al (2012) Antiangiogenic agents increase breast cancer stem cell via the generation of tumor hypoxia. Proc Natl Acad Sci U S A 109:2784–2789

Conrotto P, Valdembri D, Corso S et al (2005) Sema 4D induces angiogenesis through Met recruitment by plexin B1. Blood 105:4321–4328

Cormier SA, Taranova AG, Bedient C et al (2006) Pivotal advance: eosinophil infiltration of solid tumors in an early and persistent inflammatory host response. J Leukoc Biol 79:1131–1139

Corthay A (2014) Does the immune system naturally protect against cancer? Front Immunol 12:197

Coussens LM, Werb Z (1996) Matrix metalloproteinases and the development of cancer. Chem Biol 3:895–904

Coussens LM, Raymond WW, Bergers G et al (1999) Inflammatory mast cells up-regulate angiogenesis during squamous epithelial carcinogenesis. Gene Dev 13:1382–1397

Coussens LM, Tinkle CL, Hanahan D et al (2000) MMP-9 supplied by bone marrow–derived cells contributes to skin carcinogenesis. Cell 103:481–490

Curiel TJ, Cheng P, Mottram P et al (2004) Dendritic cell subsets differentially regulate angiogenesis in human ovarian cancer. Cancer Res 64:5535–5538

Danelli L, Frossi B, Gri G et al (2004) Mast cells boost myeloid-derived suppressor cell activity and contribute to the development of tumor-favoring microenvironment. Cancer Immunol Res 3:85–95

Das A, Sinha M, Datta S et al (2015) Monocyte and macrophage plasticity in tissue repair and regeneration. Am J Pathol 185:2596–2606

De Luisi A, Mangialardi G, Ria R et al (2009) Antiangiogenic activity of carebastine: a plausible mechanism affecting airway remodelling. Eur Respir J 34:958–966

De Nardo DG, Barreto JB, Andreu P et al (2009) CD4+ T cells regulate pulmonary metastasis of mammary carcinomas by enhancing protumor properties of macrophages. Cancer Cell 16:91–102

De Palma M, Lewis CE (2013) Macrophage regulation of tumor responses to anticancer therapies. Cancer Cell 23:277–286

De Palma M, Naldini L (2009) Tie-2 expressing monocytes (TEMs): novel targets and vehicles of anticancer therapy ? Biochim Biophys Acta 1796:5–10

De Palma M, Venneri MA, Roca C et al (2003) Targeting exogenous genes to tumor angiogenesis by transplantation of genetically modified hematopoietic stem cells. Nat Med 9:789–795

De Palma M, Venneri MA, Galli R (2005) Tie2 identifies a hematopoietic lineage of proangiogenic monocytes required for tumor vessel formation and a mesenchymal pouplation of pericyte progenitors. Cencer Cell 8:211–226

De Palma M, Mazzieri R, Politi LS et al (2008) Tumor-targeted interferon alpha delivery by Tie2-expressing monocytes inhibits tumor growth and metastasis. Cencer Cell 14:299–311

de Paulis A, Prevete N, Fiorentino I et al (2006) Expression and functions of the vascular endothelial growth factors and their receptors in human basophils. J Immunol 177:7322–7331

de Souza DA, Toso VD, Campos MRdC et al (2012) Expression of mast cell proteases correlates with mast cell maturation and angiogenesis during tumor progression. PLoS One 7:e40790

de Visser KE, Korets LV, Coussens LM (2005) De novo carcinogenesis promoted by chronic inflammation is B lymphocyte dependent. Cancer Cell 7:411–423

De Wever O, Van Bockstal M, Mareel M et al (2014) Carcinoma-associated fibroblasts provide operational flexibility in metastasis. Semin Cancer Biol 25:33–46

Deligdisch L, Jacobs AJ, Cohen CJ (1982) Histologic correlates of virulence in ovarian adenocarcinoma. II. Morphologic correlates of host response. Am J Obstet Gynecol 144:885–889

DeNardo DG, Brennan DJ, Rexhepaj E et al (2011) Leukocyte complexity predicts breast cancer survival and functionally regulates response to chemotherapy. Cancer Discov 1:54–67

Deng X, Tolstanova G, Khomenko T et al (2009) Mesalamine restores angiogenic balance in experimental ulcerative colitis by reducing expression of endostatin and angiostatin: novel molecular mechanism for therapeutic action of mesalamine. J Pharmacol Exp Ther 331:1071–1078

Denhardt DT, Noda M, O'Regan AW et al (2001) Osteopontin as a means to cope with environmental insults: regulation of inflammation, tissue remodeling, and cell survival. J Clin Invest 107:1055–1061

Desgrosselier JS, Cheres DA (2010) Integrins in cancer: biological implications and therapeutic opportunities. Nat Rev Cancer 10:9–22

Detmar M, Brown LF, Schön MP et al (1998) Increased microvascular density and enhanced leukocyte rolling and adhesion in the skin of VEGF transgenic mice. J Invest Dermatol 111:1–6

Detoraki A, Staiano RI, Granata F et al (2009) Vascular endothelial growth factors synthesized by human lung mast cells exert angiogenic effects. J Allergy Clin Immun 123:1142–1149. e1145

Devalaraja RM, Nanney LB, Qian Q et al (2000) Delayed wound healing in CXCR2 knockout mice. J Invest Dermatol 115:234–244

Dhodapkar MV (2005) Immune response to premalignancy: insights from patients with monoclonal gammopathy. Ann N Y Acad Sci 1062:22–28

Dhodapkar MV, Krasovsky J, Osman K et al (2003) Vigorous premalignancy-specific effector T cell response in the bone marrow of patients with monoclonal gammopathy. J Exp Med 198:1753–1757

Dias S, Boyd R, Balkwill F (1998) IL-12 regulates VEGF and MMPs in a murine breast cancer model. Int J Cancer 78:361–365

Dighe A, Richards E, Old L et al (1994) Enhanced in vivo growth and resistance to rejection of tumor cells expressing dominant negative IFN-greceptors. Immunity 1:447–456

Dineen SP, Lynn KD, Holloway SE et al (2008) Vascular endothelial growth factor receptor 2 mediates macrophage infiltration into orthotopic pancreatic tumors in mice. Cancer Res 68:4340–4346

Di Pietro LA, Polverini PJ (1993) Angiogenic macrophages produce the angiogenic inhibitor thrombospondin-1. Am J Pathol 143:678–684

Doroshow JH, Gaur S, Markel S et al (2013) Effects of iodonium-class flavin dehydrogenase inhibitors on growth, reactive oxygen production, cell cycle progression, NADPH oxidase 1 levels, and gene expression in human colon cancer cells and xenografts. Free Radic Biol Med 57:162–175

Dorsch M, Hock H, Kunzendorf U et al (1993) Macrophage colony-stimulating factor gene transfer into tumor cells induces macrophage infiltration but not tumor suppression. Eur J Immunol 23:186–190

Dubravec DB, Spriggs DR, Mannick JA et al (1990) Circulating human peripheral blood granulocytes synthesize and secrete tumor necrosis factor alpha. Proc Natl Acad Sci U S A 87:6758–6761

Dudas J, Fullar A, Romani A et al (2013) Curcumin targets fibroblast-tumor cell interactions in oral squamous cell carcinoma. Exp Cell Res 319:800–809

Dunn GP, Bruce AT, Ikeda H et al (2002) Cancer immunoediting: from immunosurveillance to tumor escape. Nat Immunol 3:991–998

Dunn GP, Old LJ, Schreiber RD (2004) The three Es of cancer immunoediting. Annu Rev Immunol 22:329–360

Dvorak AM (1989) Human mast cells. In: Beck F et al (eds) Advances in anatomy embryology and cell biology. Srpinger, Berlin

Dvorak AM, Mihm MC, Osage JE et al (1980) Melanoma. An ultrastructural study of the host inflammatory and vascular responses. J Invest Dermatol 75:388–393

Eberlein C, Kendrew J, McDaid K et al (2013) A human monoclonal antibody 264RAD targeting αvß6 integrin reduces tumour growth and metastasis, and modulates key biomarkers in vivo. Oncogene 32:4406–4416

Ebos JML, Kerbel RS (2011) Antiangiogenic therapy: impact on invasion, disease progression, and metastasis. Nat Rev Clin Oncol 8:210–221

Ehrlich P (1878) Beitrage zur Theorie und Praxis der histologischen Farbung; 1878. Thesis. Leipzig University

Ehrlich P (1909) Ueber den jetzigen Stand der Karzinomforschung. Ned Tijdschr Geneeskd 5:273–290

Eklund KK (2007) Mast cells in the pathogenesis of rheumatic diseases and as potential targets for anti-rheumatic therapy. Immunol Rev 217:38–52

Elpek GO, Gelen T, Aksoy NH et al (2001) The prognostic relevance of angiogenesis and mast cells in squamous cell carcinoma of the oesophagus. J Clin Pathol 54:940–944

Elsheikh E, Uzunel M, He Z et al (2005) Only a specific subset of human peripheral-blood monocytes has endothelial-like functional capacity. Blood 106:2347–2355

Engels EA, Frisch M, Goedert JJ et al (2002) Merkel cell carcinoma and HIV infection. Lancet 359:497–498

Epstein NA, Fatti LP (1976) Prostatic carcinoma: some morphological features affecting prognosis. Cancer 37:2455–2465

Erez N, Truitt M, Olson P et al (2010) Cancer-associated fibroblasts are activated in incipient neoplasia to orchestrate tumor-promoting inflammation in NF-kappaB-dependent manner. Cancer Cell 17:135–147

Ericos R, Cybilos S, Aravena R et al (2017) Diabetic concentrations of metformin inhibit platelet-mediated ovarian cancer cell progression. Oncotarget 8:20865–20880

Escudier B, Porta C, Bono P et al (2014) Randomized, controlled, double-blind, cross-over trial assessing treatment preference for pazopanib versus sunitinib in patients with metastatic renal cell carcinoma: PISCES Study. J Clin Oncol 32:1412–1418

Evans R (1977a) Effects of X-irradiaton on host cell infiltration and growth of murine fibrosarcoma. Br J Cancer 35:557–566

Evans R (1977b) The effect of azathioprine on host-cell infiltration and growth of a murine fibrosarcoma. Int J Cancer 20:120–128

Facciabene A, Motz GT, Coukos G (2012) T regulatory cells: key players in tumor immune escape and angiogenesis. Cancer Res 72:2162–2171

Fangradt M (2012) Human monocytes and macrophages differ in their mechanisms of adaptation to hypoxia. Arthritis Res Ther 14:R181

Feijoo E, Alfaro C, Mazzolini G et al (2005) Dendritic cells delivered inside human carcinomas are sequestered by interleukin-8. Int J Cancer 116:275–281

Feistritzer C, Kaneider NC, Sturn DH et al (2004) Expression and function of the vascular endothelial growth factor receptor FLT-1 in human eosinophils. Am J Resp Cell Mol 30:729–735

Feng W, Madajka M, Kerr BA et al (2011) A novel role for platelet secretion in angiogenesis: mediating bone marrow-derived cell mobilization and homing. Blood 117:3893–3902

Fernandez Pujol B, Lucibello FC, Gehling UM et al (2000) Endothelial-like cells derived from human CD14 positive monocytes. Differentiation 65:287–300

Fidler IJ (1986) Rationale and methods for the use of nude mice to study the biology and therapy of human cancer metastasis. Cancer Metastasis Rev 5:29–49

Fischer-Colbrie R, Kirchmair R, Kahler C et al (2005) Secretoneurin: a new player in angiogenesis and chemotaxis linking nerves, blood vessels and the immune system. Curr Protein Pept Sci 6:373–385

Fitzsimons C, Molinari B, Duran H et al (1997) Atypical association of H 1 and H 2 histamine receptors with signal transduction pathways during multistage mouse skin carcinogenesis. Inflamm Res 46:292–298

Foley EJ (1953) Antigenic properties of methylcholantherene-induced tumors in mice of the strain of origin. Cancer Res 13:835

Franco OE, Shaw AK, Strand DW et al (2010) Cancer associated fibroblasts in cancer pathogenesis. Semin Cell Dev Biol 21:33–39

Fridlender ZG, Sun J, Kim S et al (2009) Polarization of tumor-associated neutrophil phenotype by TGF-beta: N1 versus N2 TAN. Cancer Cell 16:183–194

Fujiyama S, Amano K, Uehira K et al (2003) Bone marrow monocyte lineage cells adhere on injured endothelium in a monocyte chemoattractant protein-1-dependent manner and accelerate reendothelialization as endothelial progenitor cells. Circ Res 93:980–989

Fukumura D, Xavier R, Sugiura T et al (1998) Tumor induction of VEGF promoter activity in stromal cells. Cell 94:715–725

Fukushima N, Satoh T, Sano M et al (2001) Angiogenesis and mast cells in non-hodgkin's lymphoma: a strong correlation in angioimmunoblastic T-cell lymphoma. Leuk Lymphoma 42:709–720

Fulop T, Kotb R, Fortin CF et al (2010) Potential role of immunosenescence in cancer development. Ann N Y Acad Sci 1197:158–165

Gabbiani G, Ryan GB, Majno G (1971) Presence of modified fibroblasts in granulation tissue and their possible role in wound contraction. Experientia 27:549–550

Gabrilovich DJ, Nagaraj S (2009) Myeloid-derived suppressor cells as regulators of the immune system. Nat Rev Immunol 9:162–174

Gabrilovich D, Ishida T, Oyama T et al (1998) Vascular endothelial growth factor inhibits the development of dendritic cells and dramatically affects the differentiation of multiple hematopoietic lineages in vivo. Blood 92:4150–4166

Gabrilovich DI, Ostrand-Rosenberg S, Bronte V (2012) Coordinated regulation of myeloid cells by tumours. Nat Rev Immunol 12:253–268

Gaidano G, Dalla-Favera R (1992) Biologic aspects of human immunodeficiency virus-related lymphoma. Curr Opin Oncol 4:900–906

Galli SJ, Metcalfe DD, Dvorak AM (2001) Basophils and mast cells and their disorders. In: Beutler E et al (eds) Williams Hematology, vol 1. Mc-Graw-Hill, New York

Gao D, Nolan DJ, Mellick AS, Bambino K et al (2008) Endothelial progenitor cells control the angiogenic switch in mouse lung metastasis. Science 319:195–198

Garg K, Sell SA, Madurantakam P et al (2009) Angiogenic potential of human macrophages on electrospun bioresorbable vascular grafts. Biomed Mater 4:031001

Gasser S, Raulet DH (2006) The DNA damage response arouses the immune system. Cancer Res 66:3959–3962

Geissmann F, Manz MG, Jung S et al (2010) Development of monocytes, macrophages, and dendritic cells. Science 327:656–661

Ghosh N, Chaki R, Mandal SC (2010) COX-2 as a target for cancer chemotherapy. Pharmacol Rep 62:233–244

Giannoni E, Bianchini F, Masieri L et al (2010) Reciprocal activation of prostate cancer cells and cancer-associated fibroblasts stimulates epithelial-mesenchymal transition and cancer stemness. Cancer Res 70:6945–6956

Gibbs BF (2005) Human basophils as effectors and immunomodulators of allergic inflammation and innate immunity. Clin Exp Med 5:43–49

Giraudo E, Inoue M, Hanahan D (2004) An amino-bisphosphonate targets MMP-9–expressing macrophages and angiogenesis to impair cervical carcinogenesis. J Clin Invest 114:623–633

Gleave ME, Elhilali M, Fradet Y et al (1998) Interferon γ-1b compared with placebo in metastatic renal-cell carcinoma. Canadian Urologic Oncology Group N Engl J Med 338:1265–1271

Glover LE, Colgan SP (2011) Hypoxia and metabolic factors that influence IBD pathogenesis. Gastroenterology 140:1748–1755

Glowacki J, Mulliken JB (1982) Mast cells in hemangiomas and vascular malformations. Pediatrics 70:48–51

Goede V, Brogelli L, Ziche M et al (1999) Induction of inflammatory angiogenesis by monocyte chemoattractant protein-1. Int J Cancer 82:765–770

Gordon-Weeks AN, Lim SY, Yuzhalin AE et al (2017) Neutrophils promote hepatic metastasis growth through fibroblast growth factor-2 dependent angiogenesis. Hepatology 65:1920–1935

Gottfried E, Kreutz M, Haffner S et al (2007) Differentiation of human tumour-associated dendritic cells into endothelial-like cells: an alternative pathway of tumour angiogenesis. Scand J Immunol 65:329–335

Gotthardt D, Putz EM, Grundschober E et al (2016) STAT5 is a key regulator in NK cells and acts as a molecular switch from tumor surveillance to tumor promotion. Cancer Discov 6:414–429

Gounaris E, Erdman SE, Restaino C et al (2007) Mast cells are an essential hematopoietic component for polyp development. Proc Natl Acad Sci U S A 104:19977–19982

Graham RM, Graham JB (1966) Mast cells and cancer of the cervix. Surgery, Gynecol Obstet 123:3–9

Graves DT, Valente AJ (1991) Monocyte chemotactic proteins from human tumor cells. Biochem Pharmacol 41:333–337

Greene HS, Harvey EK (1964) The relationship between the dissemination of tumor cells and the distribution of metastases. Cancer Res 24:799–811

Greenhough A, Smartt HJM, Moore AE et al (2009) The COX-2/PGE2 pathway: key roles in the hallmarks of cancer and adaptation to the tumour microenvironment. Carcinogenesis 30:377–386

Grenier A, Chollet-Martin S, Crestani B et al (2002) Presence of a mobilizable intracellular pool of hepatocyte growth factor in human polymorphonuclear neutrophils. Blood 99:2997–3004

Grimbaldeston MA, Nakae S, Kalesnikoff J et al (2007) Mast cell-derived interleukin 10 limits skin pathology in contact dermatitis and chronic irradiation with ultraviolet B. Nat Immunol 8:1095–1104

Groneberg DA, Bester C, Grützkau A et al (2005) Mast cells and vasculature in atopic dermatitis - potential stimulus of neoangiogenesis. Allergy 60:90–97

Gross L (1943) Intradermal immunization of C3H mice against a sarcoma that originated in an animal of the same line. Cancer Res 3:326

Gruber BL, Marchese MJ, Kew R (1995) Angiogenic factors stimulate mast-cell migration. Blood 86:2488–2493

Grutzkau A, Kruger-Krasagakes S, Baumeister H et al (1998) Synthesis, storage, and release of vascular endothelial growth factor/vascular permeability factor (VEGF/VPF) by human mast cells: implications for the biological significance of VEGF206. Mol Biol Cell 9:875–884

Guba M, von Breitenbuch P, Steinbauer M et al (2002) Rapamycin inhibits primary and metastatic tumor growth by antiangiogenesis: involvement of vascular endothelial growth factor. Nat Med 8:128–135

Guiducci C, Vicari AP, Sangaletti S et al (2005) Redirecting in vivo elicited tumor infiltrating macrophages and dendritic cells towards tumor rejection. Cancer Res 65:3437–3446

Gulley JL, Mulders P, Albers P et al (2015) Perspectives on sipuleucel-T: its role in the prostate cancer treatment paradigm. Oncoimmunology 10:e1107698

Gutschalk CM, Herold-Mende CC, Fusenig NE et al (2006) Granulocyte colony-stimulating factor and granulocyte-macrophage colony-stimulating factor promote malignant growth of cells from head and neck squamous cell carcinomas in vivo. Cancer Res 66:8026–8036

Hanada T, Nakagawa M, Emoto A et al (2000) Prognostic value of tumor-associated macrophage count in human bladder cancer. Int J Urol 7:263–269

Hanahan D, Folkman J (1996) Patterns and emerging mechanisms of the angiogenic switch during tumorigenesis. Cell 86:353–364

Hanahan D, Weinberg RA (2011) Hallmarks of cancer: the next generation. Cell 144:646–674

Hartveit F (1981) Mast cells and metachromasia in human breast cancer: their occurrence, significance and consequence: a preliminary report. J Pathol 134:7–11

Hattori K, Dias S, Heissig B et al (2001) Vascular endothelial growth factor and angiopoietin-1 stimulate postnatal hematopoiesis by recruitment of vasculogenic and hematopoietic stem cells. J Exp Med 193:1005–1014

Hayahawa Y, Smyth MJ (2006) NKG2D and cytotoxic effector function in tumor immune surveillance. Semin Immunol 18:176–185

He YF, Zhang GM, Wang XH et al (2004) Blocking programmed death-1 ligand-PD-1 interactions by local gene therapy results in enhancement of antitumor effect of secondary lymphoid tissue chemokine. J Immunol 173:4919–4928

Heike Y, Sone S, Yano S et al (1993) M-CSF gene transduction in multidrug-resistant human cancer cells to enhance anti-P-glycoprotein antibody-dependent macrophage-mediated cytotoxicity. Int J Cancer 54:851–857

Hill RP, Marie-Egyptienne DT, Hedley DW (2009) Cancer stem cells, hypoxia and metastasis. Semin Radiat Oncol 19:106–111

Hodi FS, O'Day SJ, McDermott DF (2010) Improved survival with ipilimumab in patients with metastatic melanoma. N Engl J Med 363:711–723

Hofheinz RD, Weisser A, Willer A et al (2003) Treatment of a patient with advanced esophageal cancer with a combination of mitomycin C and capecitabine: activation of the thymidine phosphorylase as active principle? Onkologie 26:161–164

Hofstra CL, Desai PJ, Thurmond RL et al (2003) Histamine H4 receptor mediates chemotaxis and calcium mobilization of mast cells. J Pharmacol Exp Ther 305:1212–1221

Horiuchi T, Weller PF (1997) Expression of vascular endothelial growth factor by human eosinophils: upregulation by granulocyte macrophage colony-stimulating factor and interleukin-5. Am J Resp Cell Mol 17:70–77

Hoshino M, Nakamura Y, Hamid QA (2001a) Gene expression of vascular endothelial growth factor and its receptors and angiogenesis in bronchial asthma. J Allergy Clin Immunol 107:1034–1038

Hoshino M, Takahashi M, Aoike N (2001b) Expression of vascular endothelial growth factor, basic fibroblast growth factor, and angiogenin immunoreactivity in asthmatic airways and its relationship to angiogenesis. J Allergy Clin Immunol 107:295–301

Hotchkiss KA, Ashton AW, Klein RS et al (2003) Mechanisms by which tumor cells and monocytes expressing the angiogenic factor thymidine phosphorylase mediate human endothelial cell migration. Cancer Res 63:527–533

Huang B, Lei Z, Zhang GM et al (2008) SCF-mediated mast cell infiltration and activation exacerbate the inflammation and immunosuppression in tumor microenvironment. Blood 112:1269–1279

Huang Y, Yuan J, Righi E et al (2012) Vascular normalizing doses of antiangiogenic treatment reprogram the immunosuppressive tumor microenvironment and enhance immunotherapy. Proc Natl Acad Sci U S A 109:17561–17566

Hujanen ES, Terranova VP (1985) Migration of tumor cells to organ-derived chemoattractants. Cancer Res 45:3517–3521

Hussain SP, Harris CC (2007) Inflammation and cancer: an ancient link with novel potentials. Int J Cancer 121:2373–2380

Iba O, Matsubara H, Nozawa Y et al (2002) Angiogenesis by implantation of peripheral blood mononuclear cells and platelets into ischemic limbs. Circulation 106:2019–2025

Iliopoulos D (2014) MicroRNA circuits regulate the cancer inflammation link. Sci Signal 7:318

Imada A, Shijubo N, Kojima H et al (2000) Mast cells correlate with angiogenesis and poor outcome in stage I lung adenocarcinoma. Eur Respir J 15:1087

Imtiyaz HZ, Williams EP, Hickey MM et al (2010) Hypoxia-inducible factor 2α regulates macrophage function in mouse models of acute and tumor inflammation. J Clin Invest 120:2699–2714

Inoue Y, Najkayama Y, Mingawa N et al (2005) Relationship between interleukin-12-expressing cells and antigen-presenting cells in patients with colorectal cancer. Anticancer Res 25:3541–3546

Italiano JE, Richardson JL, Patel-Hett S et al (2007) Angiogenesis is regulated by a novel mechanism: pro- and antiangiogenic proteins are organized into separate platelet granules and differentially released. Blood 111:1227–1233

Izquierdo E, Canete JD, Celis E et al (2009) Immature blood vessels in rheumatoid synovium are selectively depleted in response to anti-TNF therapy. PLoS One 4:1–8

Jacobsen B, Ploug M (2008) The urokinase receptor and its structural homologue C4.4A in human cancer: expression, prognosis and pharmacological inhibition. Curr Med Chem 15:2559–2573

Jass JR (1986) Lymphocytic infiltration and survival in rectal cancer. J Clin Pathol 39:585–589

Jenkins DC, Charles IG, Thomsen LL et al (1995) Roles of nitric oxide in tumor growth. Proc Natl Acad Sci U S A 92:4392–4396

Jeong HJ, Oh HA, Nam SY et al (2013) The critical role of mast cell-derived hypoxia-inducible factor 1alpha in human and mice melanoma growth. Int J Cancer 132:2492–2501

Jett JR, Maksymiuk AW, Su JQ et al (1994) Phase III trail of recombinant interferon γ in complete responders with small-cell ling cancer. J Clin Oncol 12:2321–2326

Joseph-Silverstein J, Moscatelli D, Rifkin DB (1988) The development of a quantitative RIA for basic fibroblast growth factor using polyclonal antibodies against the 157 amino acid form of human bFGF. J Immunol Methods 110:183–192

Jurasz P, Santos-Martinez M, Radomska A et al (2006) Generation of platelet angiostatin mediated by urokinase plasminogen activator: effects on angiogenesis. J Thromb Res 4:1095–1106

Kacinski BM (1995) CSF-1 and its receptor in ovarian, endometrial and breast cancer. Ann Med 27:79–85

Kalka C, Masuda H, Takahashi T et al (2000) Transplantation of ex vivo expanded endothelial progenitor cells for therapeutic neovascularization. Proc Nat Acad Sci U S A 97:3422–3427

Kalluru R, Zeisberg M (2006) Fibroblasts in cancer. Nat Rev Cancer 6:392–401

Kaluz S, Kaluzová M, Stanbridge EJ (2008) Regulation of gene expression by hypoxia: integration of the HIF-transduced hypoxic signal at the hypoxia-responsive elements. Clin Chim Acta 395:6–13

Kamihata H, Matsubara H, Nishiue T et al (2001) Implantation of bone marrow mononuclear cells into ischemic myocardium enhances collateral perfusion and regional function via side supply of angioblasts, angiogenic ligands, and cytokines. Circulation 104:1046–1052

Kanbe N, Kurosawa M, Nagata H et al (2000) Production of fibrogenic cytokines by cord blood–derived cultured human mast cells. J Allergy Clin Immunol 106:S85–S90

Kaplan DH, Shankaran V, Dighe AS et al (1998) Demonstration of an interferon gamma-dependent tumor surveillance system in immunocompetent mice. Proc Natl Acad Sci U S A 95:7556–7561

Kerkela E, Ala-Aho R, Jeskanen L et al (2000) Expression of human macrophage metalloelastase (MMP-12) by tumor cells in skin cancer. J Invest Dermatol 114:1113–1119

Kidd S, Spaeth E, Watson K et al (2012) Origins of the tumor microenvironment: quantitative assessment of adipose-derived and bone marrowderived stroma. PLoS One 7, e30563

Kim KJ, Wang L, Su YC et al (2006) Systemic antihepatocyte growth factor monoclonal antibody therapy induces the regression of intracranial glioma xenografts. Clin Cancer Res 12:1292–1298

Kinet J-P (2007) The essential role of mast cells in orchestrating inflammation. Immunol Rev 217:5–7

Kisucka J, Butterfield CE, Duda DG et al (2006) Platelets and platelet adhesion support angiogenesis while preventing excessive hemorrhage. Proc Natl Acad Sci U S A 103:855–860

Kita H, Ohnishi T, Okubo Y et al (1991) Granulocyte/macrophage colony-stimulating factor and interleukin 3 release from human peripheral blood eosinophils and neutrophils. J Exp Med 174:745–748

Klement GL, Yip TT, Cassiola F et al (2009) Platelets actively sequester angiogenesis regulators. Blood 113:2835–2842

Klimchenko O, Di Stefano A, Geoerger B (2011) Monocytic cells derived from human embryonic stem cells and fetal liver share common differentiation pathways and homeostatic functions. Blood 117:3065–3075

Klimp AH, Hollema H, Kempinga C et al (2001) Expression of cyclooxygenase-2 and inducible nitric oxide synthase in human ovarian tumors and tumor-associated macrophages. Cancer Res 61:7305–7309

Ko JS, Zea AH, Rini BI (2009) Sunitinib mediates reversal of myeloid-derived suppressor cell accumulation in renal cell carcinoma patients. Clin Cancer Res 15:2148–2157

Koch A, Polverini P, Kunkel S et al (1992) Interleukin-8 as a macrophage-derived mediator of angiogenesis. Science 258:1798–1801

Kochne CH, Dubois RN (2004) COX-2 inhibition and colorectal cancer. Semin Oncol 31(2 suppl 7):12–21

Koide N, Nishio A, Sato T et al (2004) Significance of macrophage chemoattractant protein-1 expression and macrophage infiltration in squamous cell carcinoma of the esophagusa. Am J Gastroenterol 99:1667–1674

Kojima Y, Acar A, Eaton EN et al (2010) Autocrine TGF-beta and stromal cell-derived factor-1 (SDF-1) signaling drives the evolution of tumor-promoting mammary stromal myofibroblasts. Proc Natl Acad Sci U S A 107:20009–20014

Konno S, Eckman JA, Plunkett B (2006) Interleukin-10 and Th2 cytokines differentially regulate osteopontin expression in human monocytes and dendritic cells. J Interf Cytokine Res 26:562–567

Kopp HG, Avecilla ST, Hooper AT et al (2005) The bone marrow vascular niche: home of HSC differentiation and mobilization. Physiology 20:349–356

Koskivirta I, Rahkonen O, Mäyränpää M et al (2006) Tissue inhibitor of metalloproteinases 4 (TIMP4) is involved in inflammatory processes of human cardiovascular pathology. Histochem Cell Biol 126:335–342

Kubecova M et al (2011) Cimetidine: an anticancer drug ? Eur J Pahrm Sci 42:439–444

Kujawski M, Kortylewski M, Lee H et al (2008) Stat3 mediates myeloid cell–dependent tumor angiogenesis in mice. J Clin Invest 118:3367–3377

Kusmartsev S, Eruslanov E, Kübler H (2008) Oxidative stress regulates expression of VEGFR1 in myeloid cells: link to tumor-induced immune suppression in renal cell carcinoma. J Immunol 181:346–353

Lachter J, Stein M, Lichtig C et al (1995) Mast cells in colorectal neoplasias and premalignant disorders. Dis Colon Rectum 38:290–293

Lakshminarayanan V, Lewallen M, Frangogiannis NG et al (2001) Reactive oxygen intermediates induce monocyte chemotactic protein-1 in vascular endothelium after brief ischemia. Am J Pathol 159:1301–1311

Leali D, Dell'Era P, Stabile H et al (2003) Osteopontin (Eta-1) and fibroblast growth factor-2 cross-talk in angiogenesis. J Immunol 171:1085–1093

Ledford H (2014) Cancer treatment: the killer within. Nature 505:24–26

Lee YC, Kwak YG, Song CH (2002) Contribution of vascular endothelial growth factor to airway hyperresponsiveness and inflammation in a murine model of toluene diisocyanate-induced asthma. J Immunol 168:3595–3600

Lee CG, Link H, Baluk P et al (2004) Vascular endothelial growth factor (VEGF) induces remodeling and enhances TH2-mediated sensitization and inflammation in the lung. Nat Med 10:1095–1103

Leek RD, Lewis CE, Whitehouse R et al (1996) Association of macrophage infiltration with angiogenesis and prognosis in invasive breast carcinoma. Cancer Res 56:4625–4629

Leek RD, Landers RJ, Harris AL et al (1999) Necrosis correlates with high vascular density and focal macrophage infiltration in invasive carcinoma of the breast. Brit J Cancer 79:991–995

Leek RD, Hunt NC, Landers RJ et al (2000) Macrophage infiltration is associated with VEGF and EGFR expression in breast cancer. J Pathol 190:430–436

Leibovich SJ, Polverini PJ, Shepard HM et al (1987) Macrophage-induced angiogenesis is mediated by tumour necrosis factor-α. Nature 329:630–632

Leonard S, Murrant C, Tayade C et al (2006) Mechanisms regulating immune cell contributions to spiral artery modification – facts and hypotheses – a review. Placenta 27:40–46

Lewis JS, Landers RJ, Underwood JC et al (2000) Expression of vascular endothelial growth factor by macrophages is up-regulated in poorly vascularized areas of breast carcinomas. J Pathol 192:150–158

Lewis CE, Pollard JW (2006) Distinct role of macrophages in different tumor microenvironment. Cancer Res 66:605–612

Lewis CE, Leek RD, Harris AL et al (1994) Cytokine regulation of angiogenesis in breast tumours. Cytokine 6:581

Ley K, Laudanna C, Cybulsky MJ et al (2007) Getting to the site of inflammation: the leukocyte adhesion cascade updated. Nat Rev Immunol 7:678–689

Li X, Wilson JW (1997) Increased vascularity of the bronchial mucosa in mild asthma. Am J Respirat Crit Care 156:229–233

Lin EY, Nguyen AV, Russell RG et al (2001) Colony-stimulating factor 1 promotes progression of mammary tumors to malignancy. J Exp Med 193:727–740

Lin EY, Li JF, Gnatovskiy L et al (2006) Macrophages regulate the angiogenic switch in a mouse model of breast cancer. Cancer Res 66:11238–11246

Lin EY, J-f L, Bricard G et al (2007) Vascular endothelial growth factor restores delayed tumor progression in tumors depleted of macrophages. Mol Oncol 1:288–302

Lippert U, Möller A, Welker P (2000) Inhibition of cytokine secretion from human leukemic mast cells and basophils by H1- and H2-receptor antagonists. Exp Dermatol 9:118–124

Liss C, Fekete MJ, Hasina R et al (2001) Paracrine angiogenic loop between head-and-neck squamous-cell carcinomas and macrophages. Int J Cancer 93:781–785

Lissbrant IF, Stattin P, Wikstrom P et al (2000) Tumor associated macrophages in human prostate cancer: relation to clinicopathological variables and survival. Int J Oncol 17:445–451

Liu R, Li H, Liu L et al (2012) Fibroblast activation protein: a potential therapeutic target in cancer. Cancer Biol Ther 13:123–129

Locati M, Deuschle U, Massardi ML et al (2002) Analysis of the gene expression profile activated by the CC chemokine ligand 5/RANTES and by lipopolysaccharide in human monocytes. J Immunol 168:3557–3562

Lohela M, Casbon AJ, Olow A et al (2014) Intravital imaging reveals distinct responses of depleting dynamic tumor associated macrophage and dendritic cell subpopulations. Proc Natl Acad Sci U S A 111:E5086–E5095

Madar S, Goldstein I, Rotter V (2013) Cancer associated fibroblasts, more than meets the eye. Trends Mol Med 19:447–453

Madtes DK, Raines EW, Sakariassen KS et al (1988) Induction of transforming growth factor-α in activated human alveolar macrophages. Cell 53:285–293

Makitie T, Summanen P, Tarkkanen A et al (2001) Tumor-infiltrating macrophages (CD68+ cells) and prognosis in malignant uveal melanoma. Invest Ophthalmol Vis Sci 42:1414–1421

Mammoto T, Jiang A, Jiang E et al (2013) Platelet rich plasma extract promotes angiogenesis through the angiopoietin 1-Tie2 pathway. Microvasc Res 89:15–24

Manthey CL, Johnson DL, Illig CR et al (2009) JNJ-28312141, a novel orally active colony-stimulating factor-1 receptor/FMS-related receptor tyrosine kinase-3 receptor tyrosine kinase inhibitor with potential utility in solid tumors, bone metastases, and acute myeloid leukemia. Mol Cancer Ther 8:3151–3161

Mantovani A, Sozzani S, Locati M et al (2002) Macrophage polarization: tumor-associated macrophages as a paradigm for polarized M2 mononuclear phagocytes. Trends Immunol 23:549–555

Marimpietri D, Nico B, Vacca A et al (2005) Synregistic inhibition of human neuroblastoma-related angiogenesis by vinblastine and rapamycicn. Oncogene 24:6785–6795

Marimpietri D, Brignole C, Nico B et al (2007) Combined therapeutic effects of vinblastine and rapamycin on human neuroblastoma growth, apoptosis, and angiogenesis. Clin Cancer Res 13:3977–3988

Marinaccio C, Ingravallo G, Gaudio F et al (2014) Microvascular density, CD68 and tryptase expression in human diffuse large B-cell lymphoma. Leuk Res 38:1374–1377

Martinet Y, Bitterman PB, Mornex J-F et al (1986) Activated human monocytes express the c-sis proto-oncogene and release a mediator showing PDGF-like activity. Nature 319:158–160

Martinez C (1964) Effect of early thymectomy on development of mammary tumours in mice. Nature 203:1188

Marumo T, Schini-Kerth VB, Busse R (1999) Vascular endothelial growth factor activates nuclear factor-kappaB and induces monocyte chemoattractant protein-1 in bovine retinal endothelial cells. Diabetes 48:1131–1137

Masson V, de la Ballina LR, Munaut C et al (2005) Contribution of host MMP-2 and MMP-9 to promote tumor vascularization and invasion of malignant keratinocytes. FASEB J 19:234–236

Matsushima K, Larsen CG, DuBois GC et al (1989) Purification and characterization of a novel monocyte chemotactic and activating factor produced by a human myelomonocytic cell line. J Exp Med 169:1485–1490

Maximov A (1904) Ueber entzuendliche Veraenderungen der weissen Ratte und die dabei auftretenden Veraenderungen der Mastzellen und Fettzellen. Beitr Pathol Anat Allgem Pathol 35:93

Mazzieri R, Pucci F, Moi D et al (2011) Targeting the ANG2/TIE2 axis inhibits tumor growth and metastasis by impairing angiogenesis and disabling rebounds of proangiogenic myeloid cells. Cancer Cell 19:512–526

Mc Court M, Wang JH, Sookhai S et al (1999) Proinflammatory mediators stimulate neutrophil-directed angiogenesis. Arch Surg 134:1325–1331

Mc Ever RP (2001) Adhesive interactions of leukocytes, platelets, and the vessel wall during hemostasis and inflammation. Thromb Haemost 86:746–756

Mc Farlane GA, Munro A (1997) Helicobacter pylori and gastric cancer. Br J Surg 84:1190–1199

Melief CJM, Schwartz RS (1975) Immunocompetence and malignancy. In: Becker FF (ed) Cancer: a comprehensive treatise, vol 1. Plenum Press, New York, pp 121–160

Mesri EA, Cesarman E, Arvanitakis L et al (1996) Human herpes virus-8/Kaposi's sarcoma associated herpes virus is a new transmissible virus that infects B cells. J Exp Med 183:2385–2390

Metcalfe DD, Baram D, Mekori YA (1997) Mast cells. Physiol Rev 77:1033–1079

Mimura K, Kono K, Takahashi A et al (2006) Vascular endothelial growth factor inhibits the function of human mature dendritic cells mediated by VEGF receptor-2. Cancer Immunol Immun 56:761–770

Min B, Paul WE (2008) Basophils and type 2 immunity. Curr Opin Hematol 15:59–63

Min B, Le Gros G, Paul WE (2006) Basophils: a potential liaison between innate and adaptive immunity. Allergol Int 55:99–104

Mishra PJ, Humeniuk R, Medina DJ et al (2008) Carcinoma-associated fibroblast-like differentiation of human mesenchymal stem cells. Cancer Res 68:4331–4339

Molica S, Vacca A, Crivellato E et al (2003) Tryptase-positive mast cells predict clinical outcome of patients with early B-cell chronic lymphocytic leukemia. Eur J Hematol 71:137–139

Moller A, Lippert U, Lessmann D et al (1993) Human mast cells produce IL-8. J Immunol 151:3261–3266

Monnier Y, Zaric J, Ruegg C (2005) Inhibition of angiogenesis by non-steroidal anti-inflammatory drugs: from the bench to the bedside and back. Curr Drug Target Inflamm Allergy 4:31–38

Morrissey D, O'Sullivan GC, Tangney M (2010) Tumour targeting with systemically administered bacteria. Curr Gene Ther 10:3–14

Mostafa LK, Jones DB, Wright DH (1980a) Mechanism of the induction of angiogenesis by human neoplastic lymphoid tissue: studies on the chorioallantoic membrane (CAM) of the chick embryo. J Pathol 132:91–105

Mostafa LK, Jones DB, Wright DH (1980b) Mechanism of the induction of angiogenesis by human neoplastic lymphoid tissues: studies employing bovine aortic endothelial cells in vitro. J Pathol 132:207–216

Motzer RJ, Escudier B, Oudard S et al (2008) Efficacy of everolimus in advanced renal cell carcinoma: a doubleblind randomised, placebo-controlled phase III trial. Lancet 372:449–456

Movahedi K, Laoui D, Gysemans C et al (2010) Different tumor microenvironments contain functionally distinct subsets of macrophages derived from Ly6C(high) monocytes. Cancer Res 70:5728–5739

Mueller M (2008) Inflammation and angiogenesis: innate immune cells as modulators of tumor vascularization. In: Tumor angiogenesis. Springer, Berlin/Heidelberg, pp 351–362

Muenst S, Läubli H, Soysal SD (2016) The immune system and cancer evasion strategies: therapeutic concepts. J Intern Med 279:541–562

Muhs BE, Plitas G, Delgado Y et al (2003) Temporal expression and activation of matrix metalloproteinases-2, -9, and membrane type 1-matrix metalloproteinase following acute hindlimb ischemia. J Surg Res 111:8–15

Munitz A, Levi-Schaffer F (2004) Eosinophils: 'new' roles for 'old' cells. Allergy 59:268–275

Nacopoulou L, Azaris P, Papacharalampous N et al (1981) Prognostic significance of histologic host response in cancer of the large bowel. Cancer 47:930–936

Nahrendorf M, Swirski FK, Aikawa E et al (2007) The healing myocardium sequentially mobilizes two monocyte subsets with divergent and complementary functions. J Exp Med 204:3037–3047

Nakao S, Kuwano T, Tsutsumi-Miyahara C et al (2005) Infiltration of COX-2–expressing macrophages is a prerequisite for IL-1β–induced neovascularization and tumor growth. J Clin Invest 115:2979–2991

Nakayama T, Mutsuga N, Yao L et al (2006) Prostaglandin E2 promotes degranulation-independent release of MCP-1 from mast cells. J Leukoc Biol 79:95–104

Naldini A, Carraro F (2005) Role of inflammatory mediators in angiogenesis. Curr Drug Target Infl Allergy 4:3–8

Naldini A, Leali D, Pucci A et al (2006) Cutting edge: IL-1 mediates the proangiogenic activity of osteopontin-activated human monocytes. J Immunol 177:4267–4270

Nelson B (2010) CD20+ B cells: the other tumor-infiltrating lymphocytes. J Immunol 185:4977–4982

Nicolson GL (1988a) Cancer metastasis: tumor cell and host organ properties important in metastasis to specific secondary sites. Biochim Biophys Acta 948:175–224

Nicolson GL (1988b) Organ specificity of tumor metastasis: role of preferential adhesion, invasion and growth of malignant cells at specific secondary sites. Cancer Metastasis Rev 7:143–188

Nicolson GL, Dulski KM (1986) Organ specificity of metastatic tumor colonization is related to organ-selective growth properties of malignant cells. Int J Cancer 38:289–294

Nilsson G, Forsberg-Nilsson K, Xiang Z et al (1997) Human mast cells express functional TrkA and are a source of nerve growth factor. Eur J Immunol 27:2295–2301

Nishie A, Ono M, Shono T et al (1999) Macrophage infiltration and heme oxygenase-1 expression correlate with angiogenesis in human gliomas. Clin Cancer Res 5:1107–1113

Nishikawa H, Sakaguchi S (2010) Regulatory T cells in tumor immunity. Int J Cancer 127:759–767

Nishizuka I, Ichikawa Y, Ichikawa T et al (2001) Matrylisin stimulates DNA synthesis of cultured vascular endothelial cells and induces angiogenesis in vivo. Cancer Lett 173:175–182

Nissim Ben Efrain AH, Eli-Ashar R, Levi-Schaffer F (2010) Hypoxia modulates human eosinophil function. Clin Mol Allergy 8:10

Norrby K, Jakobsson A, Sörbo J (1986) Mast-cell-mediated angiogenesis: a novel experimental model using the rat mesentery. Virchows Arch 52:195–206

Norrby K, Jakobsson A, Sörbo J (1989) Mast-cell secretion and angiogenesis, a quantitative study in rats and mice. Virchows Arch 57:251–256

Notodihardjo PV, Morimoto N, Kakudo N et al (2015) Gelatin hydrogel impregnated with platelet rich-plasma releasate promotes angiogenesis and wound healing in murine model. J Artif Organs 1:64–71

Nowak G, Karrar A, Holmen C et al (2004) Expression of vascular endothelial growth factor receptor-2 or Tie-2 on peripheral blood cells defines functionally competent cell populations capable of reendothelialization. Circulation 110:3699–3707

Nozawa H, Chiu C, Hanahan D (2006) Infiltrating neutrophils mediate the initial angiogenic switch in a mouse model of multistage carcinogenesis. Proc Natl Acad Sci U S A 103:12493–12498

Nyberg P, Salo T, Kalluri R (2008) Tumor microenvironment and angiogenesis. Front Biosci 13:6537–6553

O'Connell RM, Rao DS, Baltimore D (2012) MicroRNA regulation of inflammatory responses. Annu Rev Immunol 30:295–312

Obermueller E, Vosseler S, Fusenig NE et al (2004) Cooperative autocrine and paracrine functions of granulocyte colony-stimulating factor and granulocyte-macrophage colony-stimulating factor in the progression of skin carcinoma cells. Cancer Res 64:7801–7812

Ogilvie BM, Hesketh PM, Rose ME (1978) Nippostrongylus brasiliensis: peripheral blood leucocyte response of rats, with special reference to basophils. Exp Parasitol 46:20–30

Ohki Y, Heissig B, Sato Y et al (2005) Granulocyte colony-stimulating factor promotes neovascularization by releasing vascular endothelial growth factor from neutrophils. FASEB J 19:2005–2007

O'Neill LA, Sheedy FJ, Mc Coy CE (2011) MicroRNAs: the fine tuners of Tool-like receptor signlling. Nat Rev Immunol 11:163–175

Orimo A, Grupta PB, Sgrol DC et al (2005) Stromal fibroblasts present in invasive human breast carcinomas promote tumor growth and angiogenesis through elevated SDF-1/CXCL12 secretion. Cell 121:335–348

Orimo A, Weinberg RA (2006) Stromal fibroblasts in cancer: a novel tumor-promoting cell type. Cell Cycle 5:1597–1601

Orsida BE, Li X, Hickey B et al (1999) Vascularity in asthmatic airways: relation to inhaled steroid dose. Thorax 54:289–295

Ostermann E, Garin-Chesa P, Heider KH et al (2008) Effective immunoconjugate therapy in cancer models targeting a serine protease of tumor fibroblasts. Clin Cancer Res 4:4584–4592

Ozao-Choy J, Ma G, Kao J et al (2009) The novel role of tyrosine kinase inhibitor in the reversal immune suppression and modulation of tumor microenvironment for immune-based cancer therapies. Cancer Res 69:2514–2522

Paget S (1889) The distribution of secondary growths in cancer of the breast. Lancet 133:571–573

Palma L, Di Lorenzo N, Guidetti B (1978) Lymphocytic infiltrates in primary glioblastomas and recidivous gliomas. Incidence, fate, and relevance to prognosis in 228 operated cases. J Neurosurg 49:854–861

Pan PY, Wang GX, Yin B et al (2007) Reversion of immune tolerance in advanced malignancy: modulation of myeloid-derived suppressor cell development by blockade of stem-cell factor function. Blood 111:219–228

Parwaresch MR (1976) The human blood basophil: morphology, origin, kinetics, function and pathology. Springer, Berlin

Pawankar R (2003) Nasal polyposis: an update: editorial review. Curr Opin Allergy Clin Immunol 3:1–6

Pawelec G, Derhov E, Larbi A (2010) Immunosenescence and cancer. Crit Rev Oncol Hematol 75:165–172

Penn I (1988) Tumors of the immunocompromised patient. Annu Rev Med 39:63–73

Pessler F, Dai L, Diaz-Torne C et al (2008) Increased angiogenesis and cellular proliferation as hallmarks of the synovium in chronic septic arthritis. Arthritis Rheum 59:1137–1146

Peterson JE et al (2012) VEGF, PF4, and PDGF are elevated in platelets of colorectal cancer patients. Angiogenesis 15:265–273

Pettipher R, Hansel TT (2008) Antagonists of the prostaglandin D2 receptor CRTH2. Drugs News Perspect 21:317–322

Philips GK, Atkins M (2015) Therapeutic uses of anti-PD-1 and anti-PD-L1 antibodies. Int Immunol 27:39–46

Pietras K, Pahler J, Bergers G et al (2008) Functions of paracrine PDGF signaling in the proangiogenic tumor stroma revealed by pharmacological targeting. PLoS Med 5:e19

Pipili-Synetos E, Papadimitriou E, Maragoudakis ME (1998) Evidence that platelets promote tube formation by endothelial cells on matrigel. Br J Pharmacol 125:1252–1257

Pittoni P, Tripodo C, Piconese S et al (2011) Mast cell targeting hampers prostate adenocarcinoma development but promotes the occurrence of highly malignant neuroendocrine cancers. Cancer Res 71:5987–5997

Polverini PJ, Leibovich SJ (1984) Induction of neovascularization in vivo and endothelial cell proliferation in vitro by tumor associated macrophages. Lab Invest 51:635–642

Polverini PJ, Leibovich SJ (1987) Effect of macrophage depletion on growth and neovascularization of hamster buccal pouch carcinomas. J Oral Pathol 16:436–441

Porta C, Riboldi E, Sica A (2011) Mechanisms linking pathogen-associated inflammation and cancer. Cancer Lett 305:250–262

Porter JF, Mitchell RG (1972) Distribution of histamine in human blood. Physiol Rev 52:361–381

Priceman S, Sung JL, Shaposhnik Z et al (2010) Targeting distinct tumor-infiltrating myeloid cells by inhibiting CSF-1 receptor: combating tumor evasion of antiangiogenic therapy. Blood 115:1451–1471

Pucci F, Venneri MA, Biziato D et al (2009) A distinguishing gene signature shared by tumor-infiltrating Tie2-expressing monocytes, blood "resident" monocytes, and embryonic macrophages suggests common functions and developmental relationships. Blood 114:901–914

Puxeddu I, Ribatti D, Crivellato E et al (2005a) Mast cells and eosinophils: a novel link between inflammation and angiogenesis in allergic diseases. J Allergy Clin Immunol 116:531–536

Puxeddu I, Alian A, Piliponsky AM et al (2005b) Human peripheral blood eosinophils induce angiogenesis. Int J Biochem Cell Biol 37:628–636

Puxeddu I, Berkman N, Nissim Ben Efraim AH et al (2009) The role of eosinophil major basic protein in angiogenesis. Allergy 64:368–374

Qian BZ, Pollard JW (2010) Macrophage diversity enhances tumor progression and metastasis. Cell 141:39–51

Qiu W, Hu M, Sridhar A et al (2008) No evidence of clonal somatic genetic alterations in cancer-associated fibroblasts from human breast and ovarian carcinomas. Nat Genet 40:650–655

Qu Z, Liebler JM, Powers MR et al (1995) Mast cells are a major source of basic fibroblast growth factor in chronic inflammation and cutaneous hemangioma. Am J Pathol 147:564–573

Qu Z, Kayton RJ, Ahmadi P et al (1998) Ultrastructural immunolocalization of basic fibroblast growth factor in mast cell secretory granules: morphological evidence for bFGF release through degranulation. J Histochem Cytochem 46:1119–1128

Queen MM, Ryan RE, Holzer RG et al (2005) Breast cancer cells stimulate neutrophils to produce oncostatin M: potential implications for tumor progression. Cancer Res 65:8896–8904

Radisky DC, Levy DD, Littlepage LE et al (2005) Rac1b and reactive oxygen species mediate MMP-3-induced EMT and genomic instability. Nature 436:123–127

Raffaghello L, Vacca A, Pistoia V et al (2014) Cancer associated fibroblasts in hematological malignancies. Oncotarget 6:2589–2603

Rak J (2010) Microparticles in cancer. Semin Thromb Hemost 36:888–906

Rappolee D, Mark D, Banda M et al (1988) Wound macrophages express TGF-alpha and other growth factors in vivo: analysis by mRNA phenotyping. Science 241:708–712

Räsänen K, Vaheri A (2010) Activation of fibroblasts in cancer stroma. Exp Cell Res 316:2713–2722

Ray PS, Fox PL (2007) A post-transcriptional pathway represses monocyte VEGF-A expression and angiogenic activity. EMBO J 26:3360–3372

Reading CL, Hutchins JF (1985) Carbohydrate structure in tumor immunity. Cancer Metastasis Rev 4:221–260

Redington AE, Roche WR, Madden J et al (2001) Basic fibroblast growth factor in asthma: Measurement in bronchoalveolar lavage fluid basally and following allergen challenge. J Allergy Clin Immunol 107:384–387

Reed JA, McNutt NS, Bogdany JK et al (2006) Expression of the mast cell growth factor interleukin-3 in melanocytic lesions correlates with an increased number of mast cells in the perilesional stroma: implications for melanoma progression. J Cutan Pathol 23:495–505

Rehman J, Li J, Orschell CM et al (2003) Peripheral blood "endothelial progenitor cells" are derived from monocyte/macrophages and secrete angiogenic growth factors. Circulation 107:1164–1169

Ren G, Dewald O, Frangogiannis NG (2003) Inflammatory mechanisms in myocardial infarction. Current Drug Targets Inflamm Allergy 2:242–256

Ribatti D (2008) Judah Folkman, a pioneer in the study of angiogenesis. Angiogenesis 11:3–10

Ribatti D (2017) The concept of immune surveillance against tumors. the first theories. Oncotarget 8:7175–7180

Ribatti D, Crivellato E (2009) The controversial role of mast cells in tumor growth. Int Rev Cell Mol Biol 275:89–131

Ribatti D, Crivellato E (2012) Mast cells, angiogenesis, and tumour growth. Biochim Biophys Acta 1822:2–8

Ribatti D, Ranieri G (2015) Tryptase, a novel angiogenic factor stored in mast cell granules. Exp Cell Res 332:157–162

Ribatti D, Vacca A (2008) Overview of angiogenesis duringtumor growth. In: Fgg WJ, Folkman J (eds) Angiogenesis. An integrative approach from science to medicine. Spinger, New York, pp 161–168

Ribatti D, Roncali L, Nico B et al (1987) Effects of exogenous heparin on the vasculogenesis of the chorioallantoic membrane. Acta Anat 130:257–263

Ribatti D, Nico B, Vacca A et al (1998) Do mast cells help to induce angiogenesis in B-cell non-Hodgkin's lymphomas? Brit J Cancer 77:1900–1906

Ribatti D, Vacca A, Nico B et al (1999) Bone marrow angiogenesis and mast cell density increase simultaneously with progression of human multiple myeloma. Br J Cancer 79:451–455

Ribatti D, Vacca A, Marzullo A et al (2000) Angiogenesis and mast cell density with tryptase activity increase simultaneously with pathological progression in B-cell non-Hodgkin's lymphomas. Int J Cancer 85:171–175

Ribatti D, Crivellato E, Candussio L et al (2001) Mast cells and their secretory granules are angiogenic in the chick embryo chorioallantoic membrane. Clin Exp Allergy 31:602–608

Ribatti D, Polimeno G, Vacca A et al (2002) Correlation of bone marrow angiogenesis and mast cells with tryptase activity in myelodysplastic syndromes. Leukemia 16:1680–1684

Ribatti D, Ennas MG, Vacca A et al (2003a) Tumor vascularity and tryptase-positive mast cells correlate with a poor prognosis in melanoma. Eur J Cancer Clin Invest 33:420–425

Ribatti D, Molica S, Vacca A et al (2003b) Tryptase-positive mast cells correlate positively with bone marrow angiogenesis in B-cell chronic lymphocytic leukemia. Leukemia 17:1428–1430

Ribatti D, Vacca A, Ria R et al (2003c) Neovascularisation, expression of fibroblast growth factor-2, and mast cells with tryptase activity increase simultaneously with pathological progression in human malignant melanoma. Eur J Cancer 39:666–674

Ribatti D, Finato N, Crivellato E et al (2005) Neovascularization and mast cells with tryptase activity increase simultaneously with pathologic progression in human endometrial cancer. Am J Obstet Gynecol 193:1961–1965

Ribatti D, Nico B, Crivellato E et al (2007) The history of the angiogenic switch concept. Leukemia 21:44–52

Ribatti D, Mangialardi G, Vacca A (2006a) Stephen Paget and the 'seed and soil' theory of metastatic dissemination. Clin Exp Med 6:145–149

Ribatti D, Nico B, Vacca A (2006b) Importance of the bone marrow microenvironment in inducing the angiogenic response in multiple myeloma. Oncogene 25:4257–4266

Ribatti D, Guidolin D, Marzullo A et al (2010) Mast cells and angiogenesis in gastric carcinoma. Int J Exp Pathol 91:350–356

Ribatti D, Ranieri G, Nico B et al (2011) Tryptase and chymase are angiogenic in vivo in the chorioallantoic membrane assay. Int J Dev Biol 55:99–102

Riboldi E, Musso T, Moroni E et al (2005) Cutting edge: proangiogenic properties of alternatively activated dendritic cells. J Immunol 175:2788–2792

Ricciardi A, Elia AR, Cappello P (2008) Transcriptome of hypoxic immature dendritic cells: modulation of chemokine/receptor expression. Mol Cancer Res 6:175–185

Richter A, Puddicombe SM, Lordan JL et al (2001) The contribution of interleukin (IL)-4 and IL-13 to the epithelial–mesenchymal trophic unit in asthma. Am J Resp Cell Mol 25:385–391

Rilke F, Colnaghi MI, Cascinelli N et al (1991) Prognostic significance of HER-2/neu expression in breast cancer and its relationship to other prognostic factors. Int J Cancer 49:44–49

Roberts NJ Jr, Prill AH, Mann TN (1986) Interleukin 1 and interleukin 1 inhibitor production by human macrophages exposed to influenza virus or respiratory syncytial virus. Respiratory syncytial virus is a potent inducer of inhibitor activity. J Exp Med 163:511–519

Rojas IG, Spencer ML, Martinez A et al (2005) Characterization of mast cell subpopulations in lip cancer. J Oral Pathol Med 34:268–273

Rolny C, Mazzone M, Tugues S et al (2011) HRG inhibits tumor growth and metastasis by inducing macrophage polarization and vessel normalization through downregulation of PlGF. Cancer Cell 19:31–44

Romagnani P, Annunziato F, Lasagni L et al (2001) Cell cycle–dependent expression of CXC chemokine receptor 3 by endothelial cells mediates angiostatic activity. J Clin Invest 107:53–63

Rosen PJ, Sweeney CJ, Park DJ et al (2010) A phase Ib study of AGM 102 in combination with bevacizumab or motesanib in patients with advanced solid tumors. Clin Cancer Res 16:2677–2687

Ross JA, Auger MJ (2002) The biology of the macrophage. In: Nurke B, Lewis CE (eds) The macrophage, 2nd edn. Oxford University Press, Oxford, pp 45–77

Ru-Chen M (2011) Epstein-Barr virus, the immune system, and associated diseases. Front Microbiol 2:5

Sablina AA, Budanov AV, Ilyinskaya GV et al (2005) The antioxidants function of the p53 tumor suppressor. Nat Med 11:1306–1313

Sabrkhany S, Griffionen AW, Oude Egbrink MG (2011) The role of blood platelets in tumor angiogenesis. Biochim Biophys Acta 1815:189–196

Salven P, Orpana A, Jonsuss H (1999) Leukocytes and platelets of patients with cancer contain high levels of vascular endothelial growth factor. Clin Cancer Res 5:487–491

Sanding H, Bulfone-paus S (2013) TLR signaling in mast cells: common and unique features. Front Immunol 3:185

Sato N, Maehara N, Goggins M (2004) Gene expression profiling of tumor-stromal interactions between pancreatic cancer cells and stromal fibroblasts. Cancer Res 64:6950–6956

Sawatsubashi M, Yamada T, Fukushima N et al (2000) Association of vascular endothelial growth factor and mast cells with angiogenesis in laryngeal squamous cell carcinoma. Virchows Arch 436:243–248

Scapini P, Nesi L, Morini M et al (2002) Generation of biologically active angiostatin kringle 1-3 by activated human neutrophils. J Immunol 168:5798–5804

Scavelli C, Di Pietro G, Cirulli T et al (2007) Zoledronic acid affects over-angiogenic phenotype of endothelial cells in patients with multiple myeloma. Mol Cancer Ther 6:3256–3262

Scavelli C, Nico B, Cirulli T et al (2008) Vasculogenic mimicry by bone marrow macrophages in patients with multiple myeloma. Oncogene 27:663–674

Schmeisser A, Garlichs CD, Zhang H et al (2001) Monocytes coexpress endothelial and macropha-gocytic lineage markers and form cord-like structures in Matrigel under angiogenic conditions. Cardiovasc Res 49:671–680

Schmeisser A, Graffy C, Daniel WG et al (2003) Phenotypic overlap between monocytes and vascular endothelial cells. Adv Exp Med Biol 522:59–74

Schruefer R, Sulyok S, Schymeinsky J et al (2006) The proangiogenic capacity of polymorpho-nuclear neutrophils delineated by microarray technique and by measurement of neovascular-ization in wounded skin of CD18-deficient mice. J Vasc Res 43:1–11

Schulz TF (2009) Cancer and viral infection in immunocompromised individuals. Int J Cancer 125:1755–1763

Schwann JB, Smyth MJ (2007) Immune surveillance of tumors. J Clin Invest 117:1137–1146

Schwartz JD, Monea S, Marcus SG et al (1998) Soluble factor(s) released from neutrophils acti-vates endothelial cell matrix metalloproteinase-2. J Surg Res 76:79–85

Scott AM, Wiseman G, Welt S et al (2003) Phase I dose-escalation study of sibrotuzumab in patients with advanced or metastatic fibroblast activation protein-positive cancer. Clin Cancer Res 9:1639–1647

Seandel M, Butler J, Lyden D et al (2008) A catalytic role for proangiogenic marrow-derived cells in tumor neovascularization. Cancer Cell 13:181–183

Seo KH, Ko H-M, Choi JH et al (2004) Essential role for platelet-activating factor-induced NF-κB activation in macrophage-derived angiogenesis. Eur J Immunol 34:2129–2137

Shamamian P, Schwartz JD, Pocock BJZ et al (2001) Activation of progelatinase A (MMP-2) by neutrophil elastase, cathepsin G, and proteinase-3: A role for inflammatory cells in tumor inva-sion and angiogenesis. J Cell Physiol 189:197–206

Shankaran V, Ikeda H, Bruce AT et al (2001) IFN gamma and lymphocytes prevent primary tumour development and shape tumour immunogenicity. Nature 410:1107–1111

Sharma P, Allison JP (2015) The future of immune check point therapy. Science 348:56–61

Shi C, Pamer EG (2011) Monocyte recruitment during infection and inflammation. Nat Rev Immunol 11:762–774

Shimoda M, Mellody KT, Orimo A (2010) Carcinoma-associated fibroblasts are a rate-limiting determinant for tumour progression. Semin Cell Dev Biol 21:19–25

Shintani S, Murohara T, Ikeda H et al (2001) Augmentation of postnatal neovascularization with autologous bone marrow transplantation. Circulation 103:897–903

Shojaei F, Wu X, Zhong C et al (2007) Bv8 regulates myeloid-cell-dependent tumour angiogen-esis. Nature 450:825–831

Shojaei F, Singh M, Thompson JD et al (2008) Role of Bv in neutrophil-dependent angiogenesis in a transgenic model of cancer progression. Proc Natl Acad Sci U S A 105:2640–2645

Shojaei F, Wu X, Qu X et al (2009) G-CSF-initiated myeloid cell mobilization and angiogenesis mediate tumor refractoriness to anti-VEGF therapy in mouse models. Proc Natl Acad Sci U S A 106:6742–6747

Shrimali RK, Yu Z, Theoret MR, Chinnasamy D et al (2010) Antiangiogenic agents can increase lymphocyte infiltration into tumor and enhance the effectiveness of adoptive immunotherapy of cancer. Cancer Res 70:6171–6180

Sica A, Schioppa T, Mantovani A et al (2006) Tumour-associated macrophages are a distinct M2 polarised population promoting tumour progression: Potential targets of anti-cancer therapy. Eur J Cancer 42:717–727

Sierko E, Wojutukiewicz MZ (2004) Platelets and angiogenesis in malignancy. Semin Thromb Hemost 30:95–108

Sierra JR, Corso S, Caione L et al (2008) Tumor angiogenesis and progression are enhanved by Sema 4D produced by tumor associated macrophages. J Exp Med 205:1673–1685

Silva J, Cerqueira F, Medeiros R (2014) Chlamydia trachomatis infection: implications for HPV status and cervical cancer. Arch Gynecol Obstet 289:715–723

Sirvastava PK (2006) Immunity to cancers. In: Male D, Brostoff J, Roth DB, Roitt I (eds) Immunology. Mosby Elsevier, 7th edition, p 422

Sluimer JC, Gasc J-M, van Wanroij JL et al (2008) Hypoxia, hypoxia-inducible transcription factor, and macrophages in human atherosclerotic plaques are correlated with intraplaque angiogenesis. J Am Coll Cardiol 51:1258–1265

Smith HW, Marshall CJ (2010) Regulation of cell signalling by uPAR. Nat Rev Mol Cell Biol 11:23–36

Solomon A, Aloe L, Pe'er J et al (1998) Nerve growth factor is preformed in and activates human peripheral blood eosinophils. J Allergy Clin Immunol 102:454–460

Sorbo J, Jakobsson A, Norrby K (1994) Mast-cell histamine is angiogenic through receptors for histamine1 and histamine2. Int J Exp Pathol 75:43–50

Soucek L, Lawlor ER, Soto D et al (2007) Mast cells are required for angiogenesis and macroscopic expansion of Myc-induced pancreatic islet tumors. Nat Med 13:1211–1218

Sozzani S, Rusnati M, Riboldi E et al (2007) Dendritic cell–endothelial cell cross-talk in angiogenesis. Trends Immunol 28:385–392

Spaeth EL, Dembinski JL, Sasser AK et al (2009) Mesenchymal stem cell transition to tumor-associated fibroblasts contributes to fibrovascular network expansion and tumor progression. PLoS One 4, e4992

Starkey JR, Crowle PK, Taubenberger S (1988) Mast-cell-deficient W/Wv mice exhibit A decreased rate of tumor angiogenesis. Int J Cancer 42:48–52

Stenzinger W, Bruggen J, Macher E et al (1982) Tumor angiogenic activity (TAA) production in vitro and growth in the nude mice by human malignant melanoma. Eur J Cancer Clin Oncol 19:649–656

Stewart T, Tsai SC, Grayson H et al (1995) Incidence of de-novo breast cancer in women chronically immunosuppressed after organ transplantation. Lancet 346:796–798

Stockmann C, Doedens A, Weidemann A et al (2008) Deletion of vascular endothelial growth factor in myeloid cells accelerates tumorigenesis. Nature 456:814–818

Strasly M, Cavallo F, Geuna M et al (2001) IL-12 inhibition of endothelial cell functions and angiogenesis depends on lymphocyte-endothelial cell cross-talk. J Immunol 166:3890–3899

Street SE, Hayakawa Y, Zhan Y et al (2004) Innate immune surveillance of spontaneous B cell lymphomas by natural killer cells and gamma delta T cells. J Exp Med 199:879–884

Stutman O (1974) Tumor development after 3-methylcholanthrene in immunologically deficient athymic-nude mice. Science 183:534–536

Stutman O (1975) Immunodepression and malignancy. Adv Cancer Res 22:261–422

Sullivan JL, Byron KS, Brewster FE et al (1980) Defcient natural killer activity in X-linked lymphoproliferative syndrome. Science 210:543–545

Sullivan R, Gans PJ, McCarroll LA (1983) The synthesis and secretion of granulocyte-monocyte colony-stimulating activity (CSA) by isolated human monocytes: kinetics of the response to bacterial endotoxin. J Immunol 130:800–807

Sun NCJ, Mc Afee WM, Hum GJ et al (1979) Hemostatic abnormalities in malignancy, a prospective study of one hundred and eight patients. Am J Clin Pathol 71:10–16

Sunderkötter C, Goebeler M, Schulze-Osthoff K et al (1991) Macrophage-derived angiogenesis factors. Pharmacol Therapeut 51:195–216

Suzuki E, Kapoor V, Jassar AS et al (2005) Gemcitabine selectively eliminates splenic Gr-1+/CD11b+ myeloid suppressor cells in tumor-bearing animals and enhances antitumor immune activity. Clin Cancer Res 11:6713–6721

Svensson C, Andersson M, Greiff L et al (1995) Exudative hyperresponsiveness of the airway microcirculation in seasonal allergic rhinitis. Clin Exp Allergy 25:942–950

Taddei ML, Cavallini L, Comito G et al (2014) Senescent stroma promotes prostate cancer progression: the role of miR-210. Mol Oncol 8:1729–1746

Takanami I, Takeuchi K, Naruke M (2000) Mast cell density is associated with angiogenesis and poor prognosis in pulmonary adenocarcinoma. Cancer 88:2686–2692

Talks KL, Tyrley H, Gatter KC et al (2000) The expression and distribution of the hypoxia-inducible factors HIF-1alpha and HIF-2 alpha in normal human tissues, cancers, and tumor-associated macrophages. Am J Pathol 157:411–421

Talmadge JE, Fidler IJ (1982) Cancer metastasis is selective or random depending on the parent tumour population. Nature 297:593–594

Talmadge JE, Donkor M, Scholar E (2007) Inflammatory cell infiltration of tumors: Jekyll or Hyde. Cancer Metastasis Rev 26:373–400

Tanaka A, Yamane Y, Matsuda H (2001) Mast cell MMP-9 production enhanced by bacterial lipopolysaccharide. J Vet Med Sci 63:811–813

Tang R, Beuvon F, Ojeda M et al (1992) M-CSF (monocyte colony stimulating factor) and M-CSF receptor expression by breast tumour cells: M-CSF mediated recruitment of tumour infiltrating monocytes? J Cell Biochem 50:350–356

Tauber AI, Chernyak L (1991) Metchnikoff and the origins of immunology: from metaphor to theory. Monographs on the history and philosophy of biology. Oxford University Press, New York, pp 1–155

Tee MK, Vigne J-L, Taylor RN (2006) All-transretinoic acid inhibits vascular endothelial growth factor expression in a cell model of neutrophil activation. Endocrinology 147:1264–1270

Teige I, Hvid H, Svensson L et al (2009) Regulatory T cells control VEGF-dependent skin inflammation. J Investig Dermatol 129:1437–1445

Temkin V, Aingorn H, Puxeddu I et al (2004) Eosinophil major basic protein: first identified natural heparanase-inhibiting protein. J Allergy Clin Immunol 113:703–709

Teng MW, Galon J, Fridman WH et al (2015) From mice to humans: developments in cancer immunoediting. J Clin Invest 125:3338–3346

Theoharides TC, Conti P (2004) Mast cells: the JEKYLL and HYDE of tumor growth. Trends Immunol 25:235–241

Tholey DM, Ahn J (2015) Impact of hepatitis C virus infection on hepatocellular carcinoma. Gastroenterol Clin N Am 44:761–773

Thomas L (1957) In: Lawrence HS (ed) Discussion of cellular and humoral aspects of hypersensitive states. Hoeber-Harper, New York, p 1959

Tomita M, Matsuzaki Y, Onitsuka T (2000) Effect of mast cells on tumor angiogenesis in lung cancer. Ann Thorac Surg 69:1686–1690

Toso JF, Gill VJ, Hwu P (2002) Phase I study of the intravenous administration of attenuated Salmonella typhi murium to patients with metastatic melanoma. J Clin Oncol 20:142–152

Toth-Jakatics R, Jimi S, Takebayashi S et al (2000) Cutaneous malignant melanoma: correlation between neovascularization and peritumor accumulation of mast cells overexpressing vascular endothelial growth factor. Hum Pathol 31:955–960

Tressel SL, Kim H, Ni CW et al (2008) Angiopoietin-2 stimulates blood flow recovery after femoral artery occlusion by inducing inflammation and arteriogenesis. Arterioscler Thromb Vasc Biol 28:1989–1995

Trinchieri G (1989) Biology of natural killer cells. Adv Immunol 47:187–376

Trinchieri G (1993) Interleukin-12 and its role in the generation of TH1 cells. Immunol Today 14:335–338

Tsuruda T, Kato J, Hatakeyama K et al (2008) Adventitial mast cells contribute to pathogenesis in the progression of abdominal aortic aneurysm. Circ Res 102:1368–1377

Tuxhorn JA, McAlhany SJ, Dang TD et al (2002) Stromal cells promote angiogenesis and growth of human prostate tumors in a differential reactive stroma (DRS) xenograft model. Cancer Res 62:3298–3307

Uccelli A, Moretta L, Pistoia V (2008) Mesenchymal stem cells in health and disease. Nat Rev Immunol 8:726–736

Ueno T, Toi M, Saji H et al (2000) Significance of macrophage chemoattractant protein-1 in macrophage recruitment, angiogenesis, and survival in human breast cancer. Clinical Cancer Res 6:3282–3289

Ulisse S, Baldini E, Sorrenti S et al (2009) The urokinase plasminogen activator system: a target for anticancer therapy. Curr Cancer Drug Targets 9:32–71

Ullrich SE, Nghiem DX, Khaskina P (2007) Suppression of an established immune response by UVA? A critical role for mast cells. Photochem Photobiol 83:1095–1100

Urbich C, Heeschen C, Aicher A et al (2003) Relevance of monocytic features for neovascularization capacity of circulating endothelial progenitor cells. Circulation 108:2511–2516

Uribe-Querol E, Rosales C (2015) Neutrophils in cancer: two sides of the same coin. J Immunol Res 2015:1–21. 983698

Vacca A, Ribatti D (2006) Bone marrow angiogenesis in multiple myeloma. Leukemia 20:193–199

Vacca A, Ribatti D, Ruco L et al (1999) Angiogenesis extent and macrophage density increase simultaneously with pathological progression in B-cellnon-Hodgkin's lymphomas. Br J Cancer 79:965–970

Van Den Berg WB, MCInnes IB (2013) Th17 cells and IL-17 A-focus on immunopathogenesis and immunotherapeutics. Semin Arthritis Rheum 43:158–170

van den Broek MW, Kägi D, Ossendorp F et al (1996) Decreased tumor surveillance in perforin-deficient mice. J Exp Med 184:1781–1790

Varney ML, Olsen KJ, Mosley RL et al (2005) Paracrine regulation of vascular endothelial growth factor-A expression during macrophage-melanoma cell interaction: role of monocyte chemotactic protein-1 and macrophage colony-stimulating factor. J Interferon Cytok Res 25:674–683

Veglia F, Gabrilovich DI (2017) Dendritic cells in cancer: the role revisited. Curr Opin Immunol 45:43–51

Vendramini-Costa JE, Carvalho JE (2012) Molecular link mechanisms between inflammation and cancer. Curr Pharm Des 18:3831–3852

Venneri MA, Palma MD, Ponzoni M et al (2007) Identification of proangiogenic TIE2-expressing monocytes (TEMs) in human peripheral blood and cancer. Blood 109:5276–5285

Verheul HMW, Hoekman K, Lupu F et al (2000a) Platelet and coagulation activation with vascular endothelial growth factor generation in soft tissue sarcomas. Clin Cancer Res 6:166–171

Verheul HMW, Jorna AS, Hoekman K et al (2000b) Vascular endothelial growth factor-stimulated endothelial cells promote adhesion and activation of platelets. Blood 96:4216–4221

Vicari AP, Caux C (2002) Chemokines in cancer. Cytokine Growth Factor Rev 13:143–154

Vink A, Schoneveld AH, Lamers D et al (2007) HIF-1alpha expression is associated with an atheromatous inflammatory plaque phenotype and upregulated in activated macrophages. Atherosclerosis 195:e69–e75

Voskas D, Babichev Y, Ling LS et al (2008) An eosinophil immune response characterizes the inflammatory skin disease observed in Tie-2 transgenic mice. J Leukoc Biol 84:59–67

Wagner EM, Sanchez J, McClintock JY et al (2008) Inflammation and ischemia-induced lung angiogenesis. Am J Phys Lung Cell Mol Phys 294:L351–L357

Waldhauer I, Steinle A (2008) NK cells and cancer immunosurveillance. Oncogene 27:5932–5943

Walsh LJ, Trinchieri G, Waldorf HA et al (1991) Human dermal mast cells contain and release tumor necrosis factor alpha, which induces endothelial leukocyte adhesion molecule 1. Proc Natl Acad Sci U S A 88:4220–4224

Watanabe M, Satoh T, Yamamoto Y et al (2008) Overproduction of IgE induces macrophage-derived chemokine (CCL22) secretion from basophils. J Immunol 181:5653–5659

Weiss L (1979) Dynamic aspects of cancer cell populations in metastasis. Am J Pathol 97:601–608

Wen J, Matsumoto K, Taniura N et al (2004) Hepatic gene expression of NK4, an HGF-antagonist/angiogenesis inhibitor, suppresses liver metastasis and invasive growth of colon cancer in mice. Cancer Gene Ther 11:419–430

White JR, Harris RA, Lee SR et al (2004) Genetic amplification of the transcriptional response to hypoxia as a novel means of identifying regulators of angiogenesis. Genomics 83:1–8

Wiesenfeld M, O'Connell MJ, Wieand HS et al (1995) Controlled clinical trial of interferon-γ as postoperative surgical adjuvant therapy for colon cancer. J Clin Oncol 13:2324–2329

Wong DT, Weller PF, Galli SJ et al (1990) Human eosinophils express transforming growth factor alpha. J Exp Med 172:673–681

Xin H, Zhang C, Herrmann A (2009) Sunitinib inhibition of Stat3 induces renal cell carcinma tumor cell apoptosis and reduces immunosuppressive cells. Cancer Res 69:2506–2513

Xue Q, Nagy JA, Manseau EJ et al (2009) Rapamycicn inhibition of the Akt/mTor pathway blocks select stages of VEGF-A 164 driven angiogenesis, in part by blocking S6kinase. Arterioscler Thromb Vasc Biol 29:1172–1178

Yamada T, Sawatsubashi M, Itoh Y et al (1998) Localization of vascular endothelial growth factor in synovial membrane mast cells: examination with "multi-labelling subtraction immunostaining". Virchows Arch 433:567–570

Yang L, DeBusk LM, Fukuda K et al (2004) Expansion of myeloid immune suppressor Gr+CD11b+ cells in tumor-bearing host directly promotes tumor angiogenesis. Cancer Cell 6:409–421

Yang Z, Zhang B, Li D et al (2010) Mast cells mobilize myeloid-derived suppressor cells in tumor microenvironment via Il-17 pathway in murine hepatocarcinoma model. PLoSONE 5:9822

Yang C, Lee H, Pal S et al (2013) B cells promote tumor progression via STAT3 regulated angiogenesis. PLoSone 8:e64159

Yano H, Kinuta M, Tateishi H et al (1999) Mast cell infiltration around gastric cancer cells correlates with tumor angiogenesis and metastasis. Gastric Cancer 2:26–32

Yao L, Sgadari C, Furuke K et al (1999) Contribution of natural killer cells to inhibition of angiogenesis by interleukin-12. Blood 93:1612–1621

Yoshimura T, Robinson EA, Tanaka S et al (1989) Purification and amino acid analysis of two human glioma-derived monocyte chemoattractants. J Exp Med 169:1449–1459

Yousefi S, Hemmann S, Weber M et al (1995) IL-8 is expressed by human peripheral blood eosinophils. Evidence for increased secretion in asthma. J Immunol 154:5481–5490

Yunis EJ, Martinez C, Smith J et al (1969) Spontaneous mammary adenocarcinoma in mice: influence of thymectomy and reconstitution with thymus grafts or spleen cells. Cancer Res 29:174–178

Zeisberg EM, Potenta S, Xie L et al (2007) Discovery of endothelial to mesenchymal transition as a source for carcinoma-associated fibroblasts. Cancer Res 67:10123–10128

Zeisberger SM, Odermatt B, Marty C et al (2006) Clodronate-liposome-mediated depletion of tumour-associated macrophages: a new and highly effective antiangiogenic therapy approach. Br J Cancer 95:272–281

Zha S, Yegnasubramanian V, Nelson WG et al (2004) Cyclooxygenase in cancer. Progress and perspectives. Cancer Lett 215:1–20

Zhang J, Chen Z, Smith GN et al (2011) Natural killer-triggered vascular transformation: maternal care before birth? Cell Mol Immunol 8:1–11

Zhang Y, Yang P, Sun T et al (2013) miRNA-126 and miNA-126 repress recruitment of mesenchymal stem cells and inflammatory monocytes to inhibit breast cancer metastasis. Nat Cell Biol 15:284–294

Zhao Y, Glesne D, Huberman E (2003) A human peripheral blood monocyte-derived subset acts as pluripotent stem cells. Proc Natl Acad Sci U S A 100:2426–2431

Ziegelhoeffer T (2004) Bone marrow-derived cells do not incorporate into the adult growing vasculature. Circ Res 94:230–238

Zielonka TM, Demkow U, Bialas B et al (2007) Modulatory effect of sera from sarcoidosis patients on mononuclear cell-induced angiogenesis. J Physiol Pharmacol 58(Suppl 5):753–766

Index

© Springer International Publishing AG 2017
D. Ribatti, *Inflammation and Angiogenesis*, https://doi.org/10.1007/978-3-319-68448-2

The manufacturer's authorised representative in the EU is Springer
Nature Customer Service Centre GmbH, Europaplatz 3, 69115 Heidelberg,
Germany. If you have any concerns regarding our products, please
contact ProductSafety@springernature.com

Printed and bound by CPI Group (UK) Ltd, Croydon, CR0 4YY

09/01/2026

02031927-0002